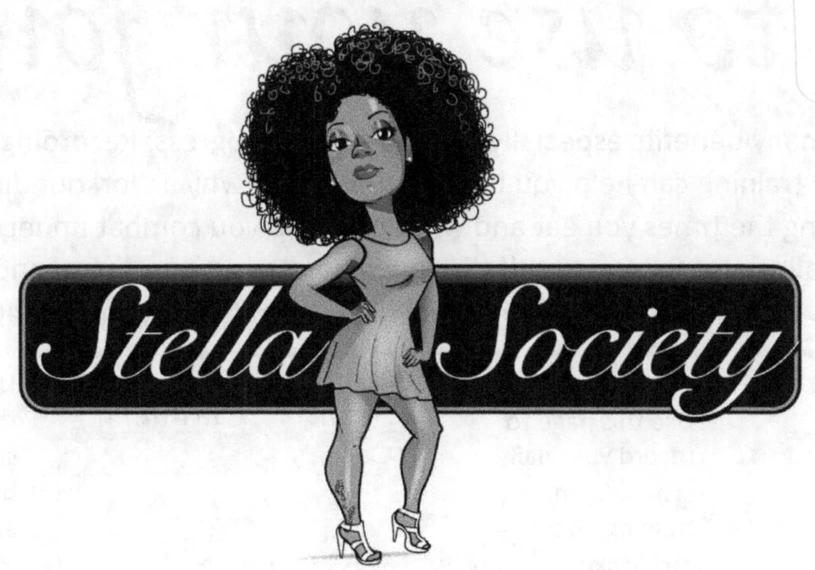

Thank you for participating in the Stella Project 2.0, a 40 day fitness confidence and nutrition challenge.
If you purchased this journal and you are not a member of the Stella Project, no worries. You can find us at stellasocietyacademy dot com, or just use it on your own 40 day fitness journey.

Always consult a physician before beginning an exercise program.

How to use your journal

Journaling has many benefits especially when tracking progress. Recording your thoughts before training can help you better understand why a workout did or didn't go too well. Recalling the times you eat and what can help you combat unnecessary cravings. Journaling also increases self-discipline, improves your mood and boost comprehension. Please use this journal to aid in your goals through your 40 days.

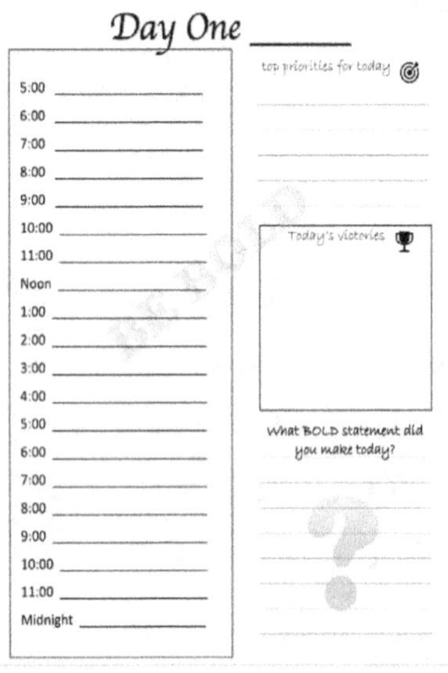

Use this page to record your daily schedule, meals, training, meetings, etc. Make sure you put the date. List your top priorities hat must be completed that day. Record your victories, like drinking all your water and reflect on the daily bestellatude

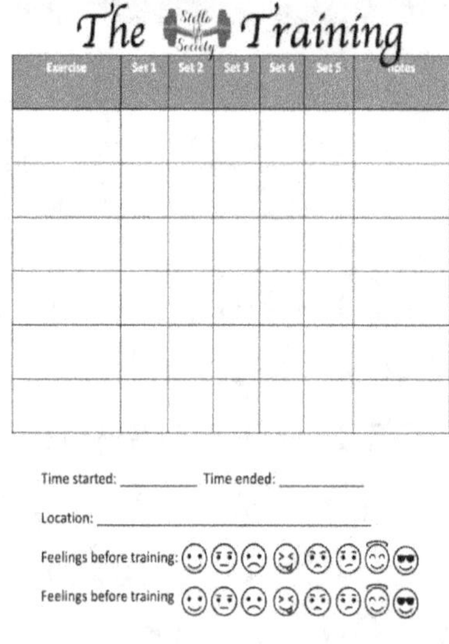

Use this page to record your training sessions. Write them down ahead of time and watch the video in case you have questions. Put the time your started and completed the training as well as how you felt before and after. Leave a note as to why you felt a certain before the training. This could effect how it went.

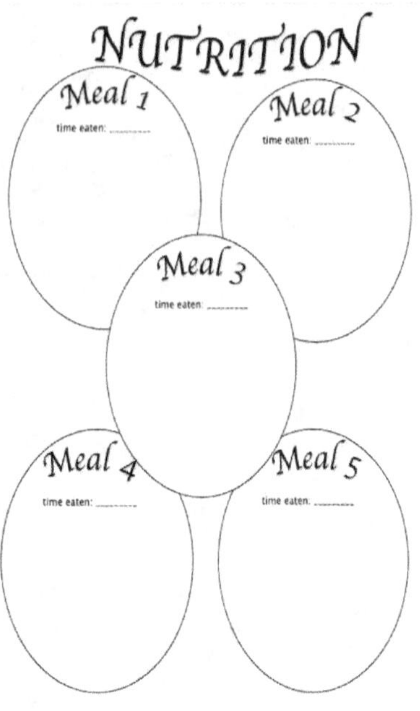

Use this page to record your meals and the time you ate them. This is important especially when tracking your progress. Try to eat your meals at the same time each day. Get your machine on a schedule so it knows how to operate its fuel.

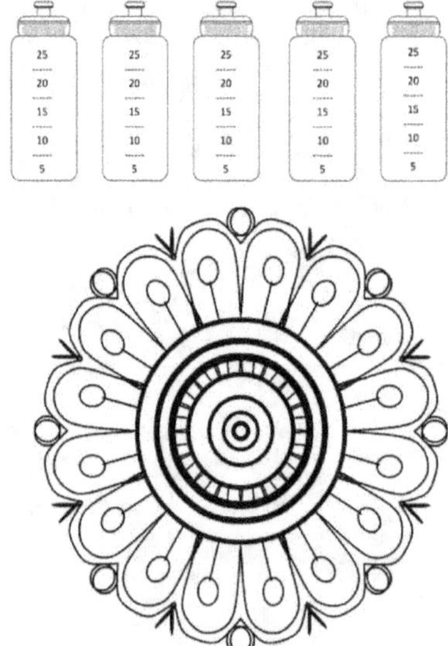

Use this page to record your water intake. Color the bottles as you complete each one. Also each hydration page has a mandala graphic to color. Coloring is a form of meditation. Choose to color this instead of reaching for something to snack on that's not you're your meal plan.

R.O.S.E.S GOAL

Rationale – why are you participating in this 40 day challenge?

____

____

Objective – what do you look to accomplish during the 40 days? What is the end game, goal?

____

____

Strategy – how will you go about completing your objective? What actions will you take.

____

____

Evaluation – how and when will you evaluate you progress? Will you use inches, weight, look, or clothes?

____

____

Schedule – create a schedule for the next 40 days. Include anything that will get in the way of your goal and find a work around.

____

____

Measurements

DATE: __________

Weight: ______

Neck ______

Shoulders ______

Chest ______

Bicep / upper arm left ________ right ______

Forearm left ________ right ______

Waist ______

Hips ______

Thighs left ________ right ______

Calf left ________ right ______

Only I Can Change My Life, No One Can Do It For Me

Day One _______

5:00 _______________________

6:00 _______________________

7:00 _______________________

8:00 _______________________

9:00 _______________________

10:00 _______________________

11:00 _______________________

Noon _______________________

1:00 _______________________

2:00 _______________________

3:00 _______________________

4:00 _______________________

5:00 _______________________

6:00 _______________________

7:00 _______________________

8:00 _______________________

9:00 _______________________

10:00 _______________________

11:00 _______________________

Midnight _______________________

____

____

____

____

Today's victories

What BOLD statement did you make today?

____

____

____

____

____

____

The Training

Exercise	Set 1	Set 2	Set 3	Set 4	Set 5	notes

Time started: _____________   Time ended: _____________

Location: ____

Feelings before training:

Feelings after training

NUTRITION

Meal 1

time eaten: _________

Meal 2

time eaten: _________

Meal 3

time eaten: _________

Meal 4

time eaten: _________

Meal 5

time eaten: _________

Hydration

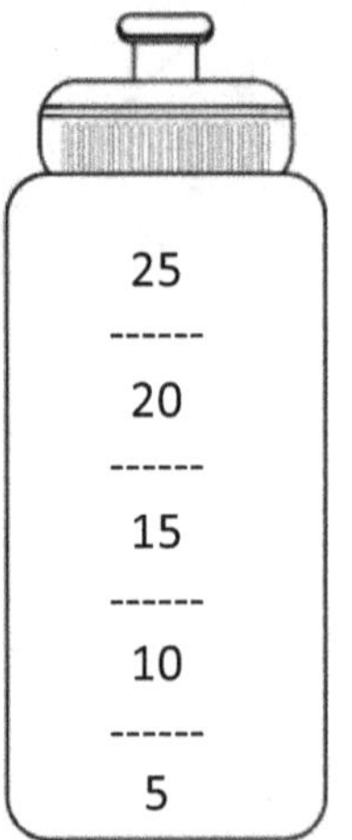

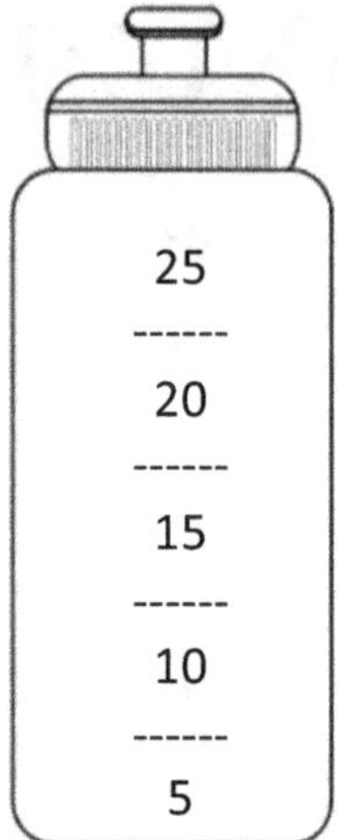

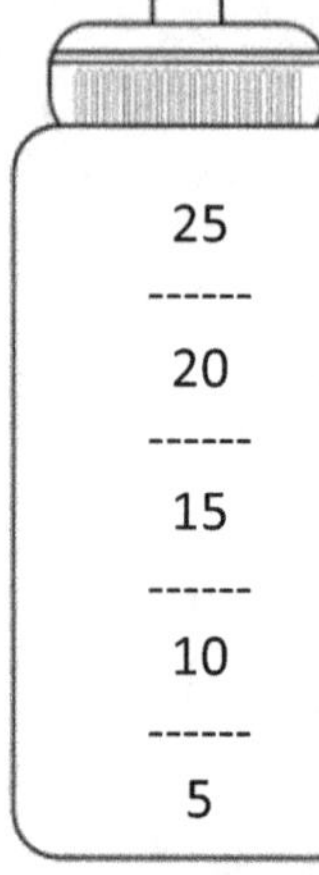

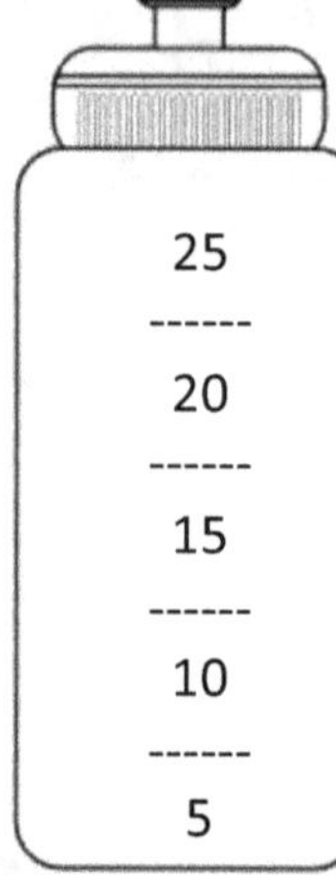

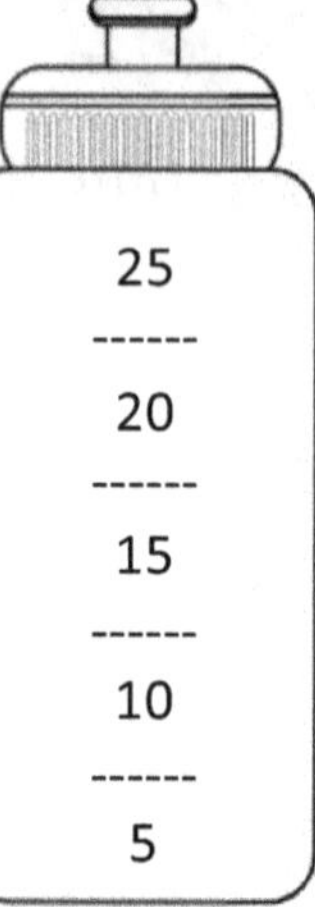

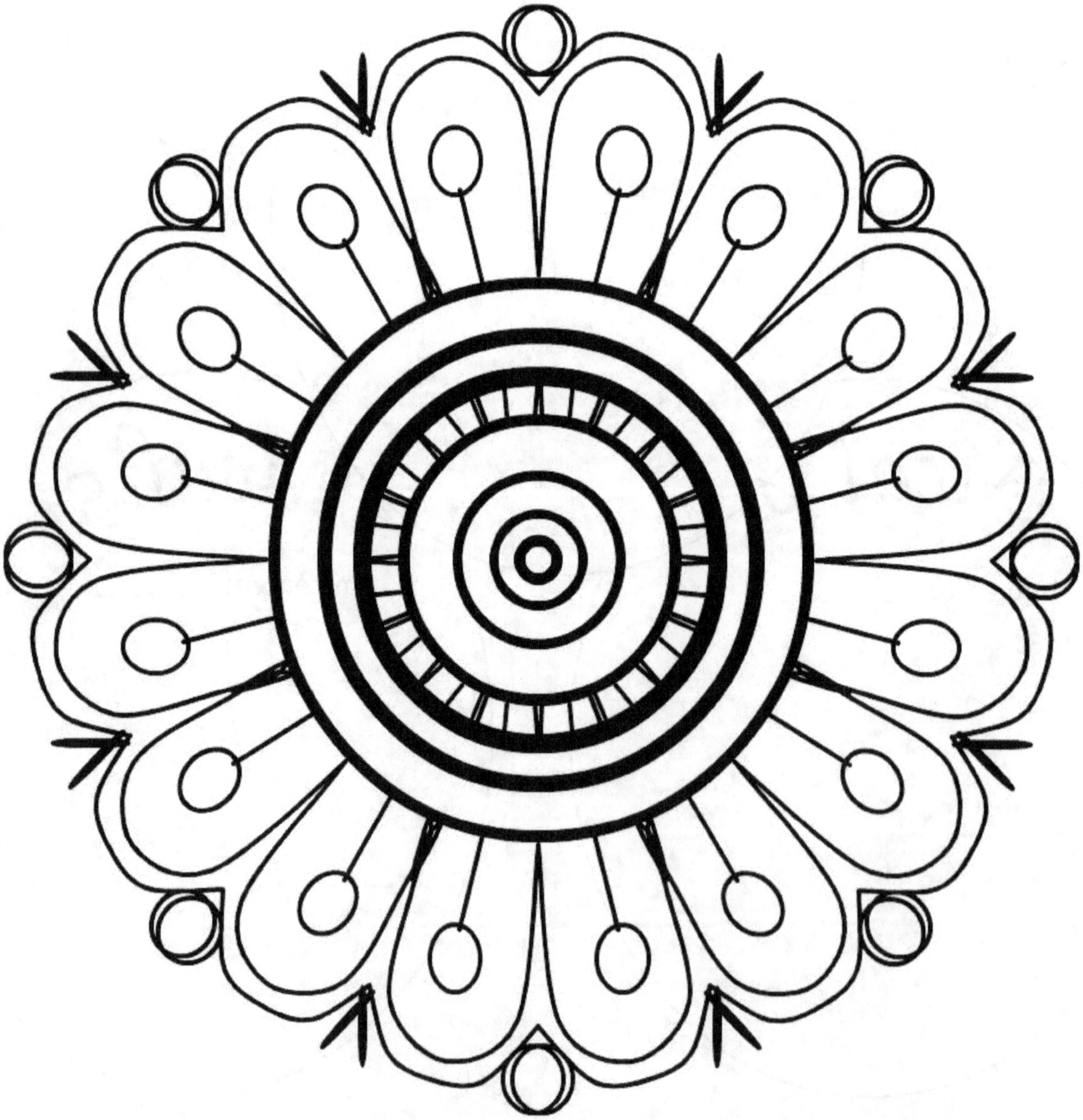

Day Two _______

5:00 _______________	

5:00 __________________

6:00 __________________

7:00 __________________

8:00 __________________

9:00 __________________

10:00 _________________

11:00 _________________

Noon __________________

1:00 __________________

2:00 __________________

3:00 __________________

4:00 __________________

5:00 __________________

6:00 __________________

7:00 __________________

8:00 __________________

9:00 __________________

10:00 _________________

11:00 _________________

Midnight _______________

top priorities for today 🎯

____

____

____

____

Today's victories 🏆

What is one thing that makes you unique??

____

____

____

____

____

____

The Training

Exercise	Set 1	Set 2	Set 3	Set 4	Set 5	notes

Time started: _______________ Time ended: _______________

Location: ____

Feelings before training:

Feelings after training

NUTRITION

Meal 1

time eaten: _________

Meal 2

time eaten: _________

Meal 3

time eaten: _________

Meal 4

time eaten: _________

Meal 5

time eaten: _________

Hydration

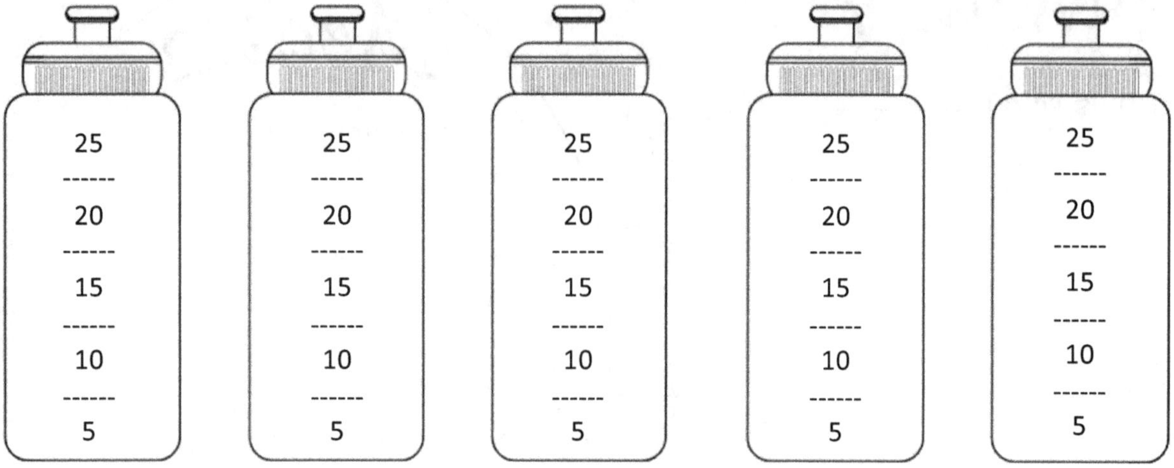

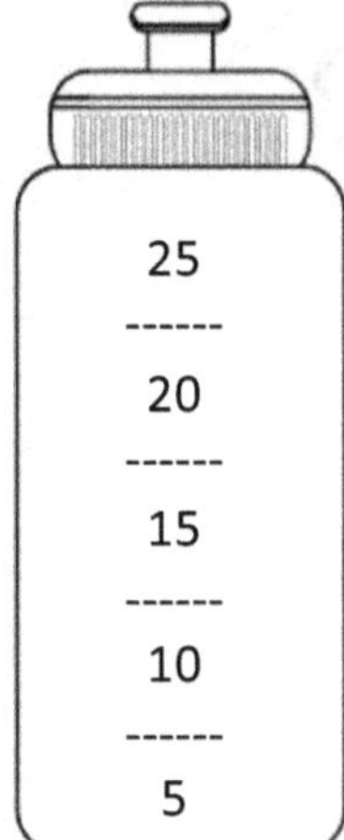
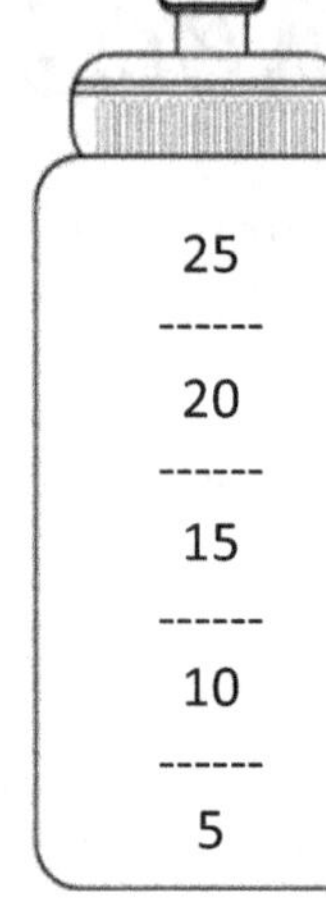
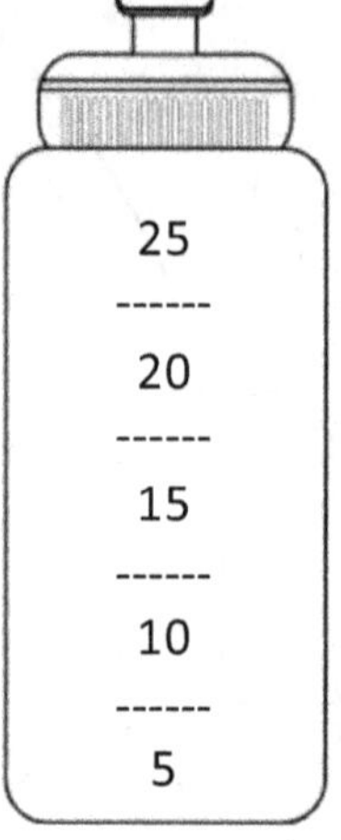

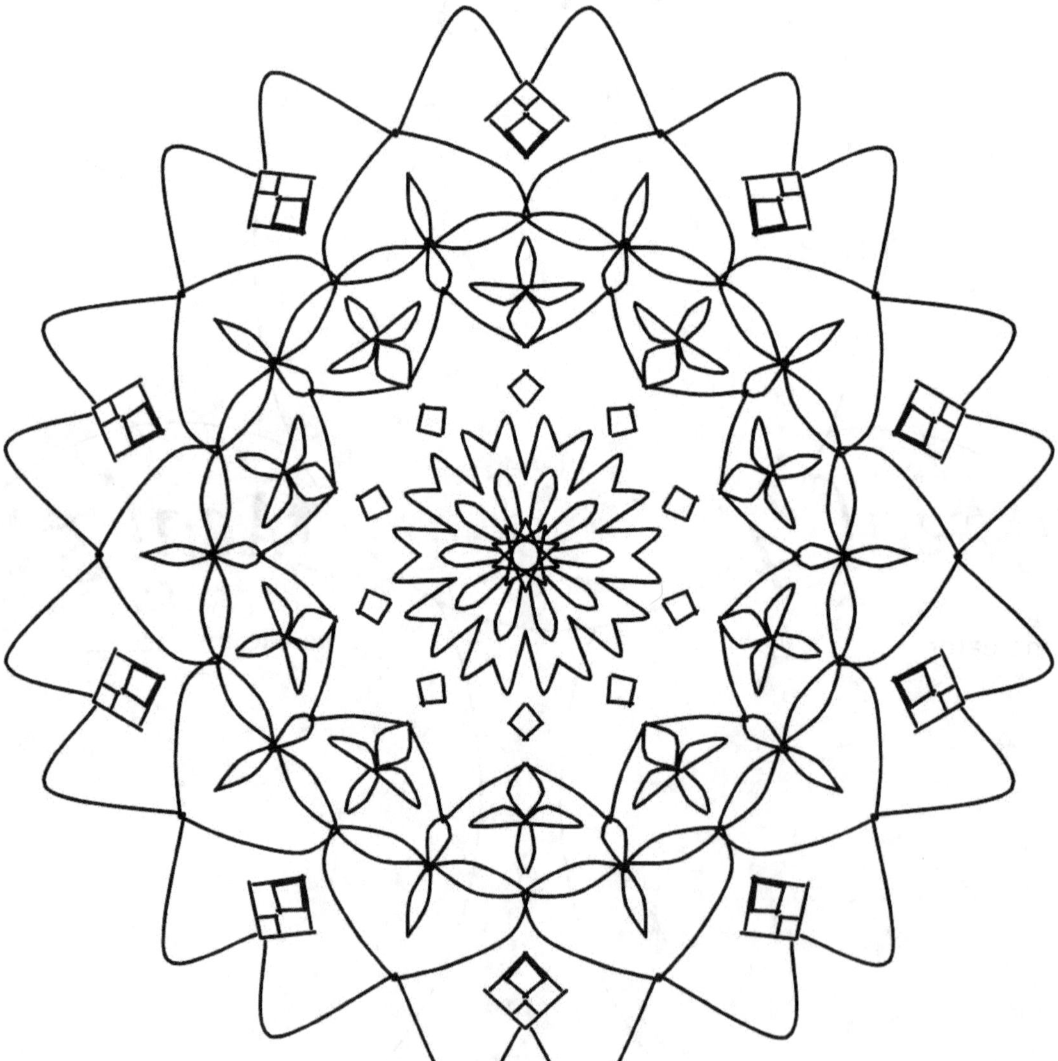

Day Three _______

5:00 _______________________

6:00 _______________________

7:00 _______________________

8:00 _______________________

9:00 _______________________

10:00 ______________________

11:00 ______________________

Noon _______________________

1:00 _______________________

2:00 _______________________

3:00 _______________________

4:00 _______________________

5:00 _______________________

6:00 _______________________

7:00 _______________________

8:00 _______________________

9:00 _______________________

10:00 ______________________

11:00 ______________________

Midnight ___________________

top priorities for today 🎯

____

____

____

____

Today's victories 🏆

What makes you brave?

____

____

____

____

____

____

The Training

Exercise	Set 1	Set 2	Set 3	Set 4	Set 5	notes

Time started: _______________   Time ended: _______________

Location: ____

Feelings before training:

Feelings after training

NUTRITION

Meal 1

time eaten: _________

Meal 2

time eaten: _________

Meal 3

time eaten: _________

Meal 4

time eaten: _________

Meal 5

time eaten: _________

Hydration

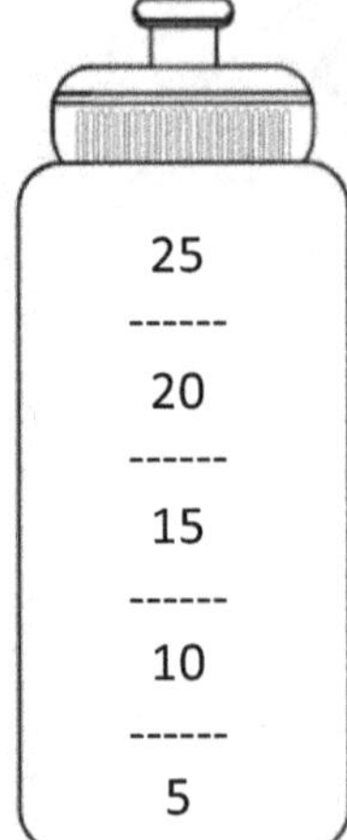 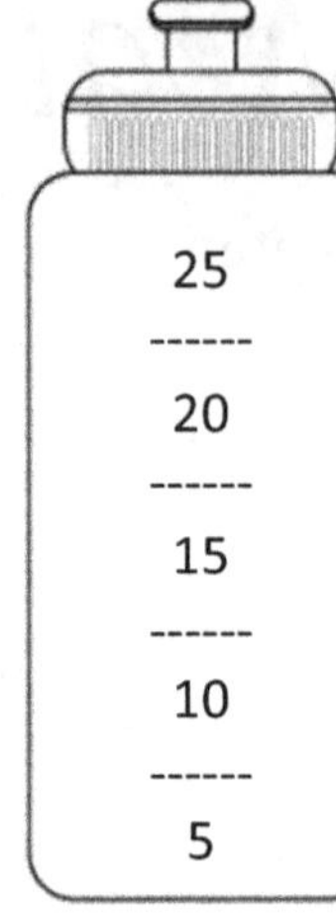 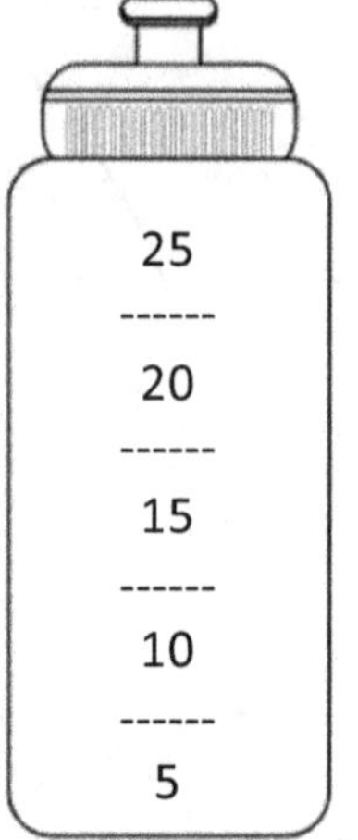 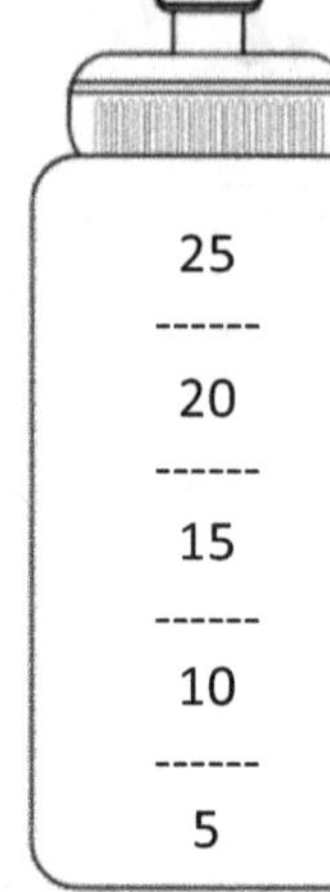 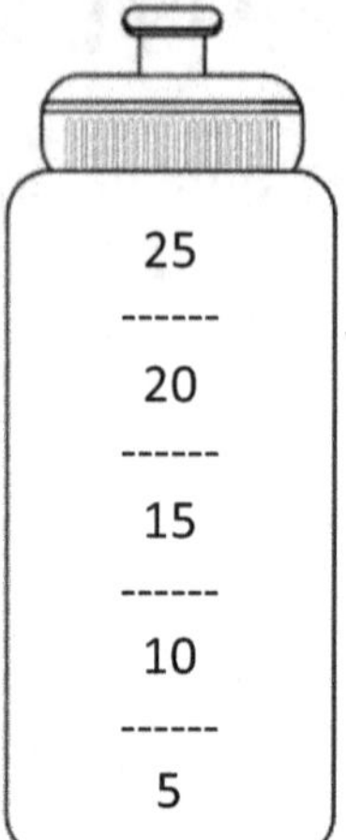

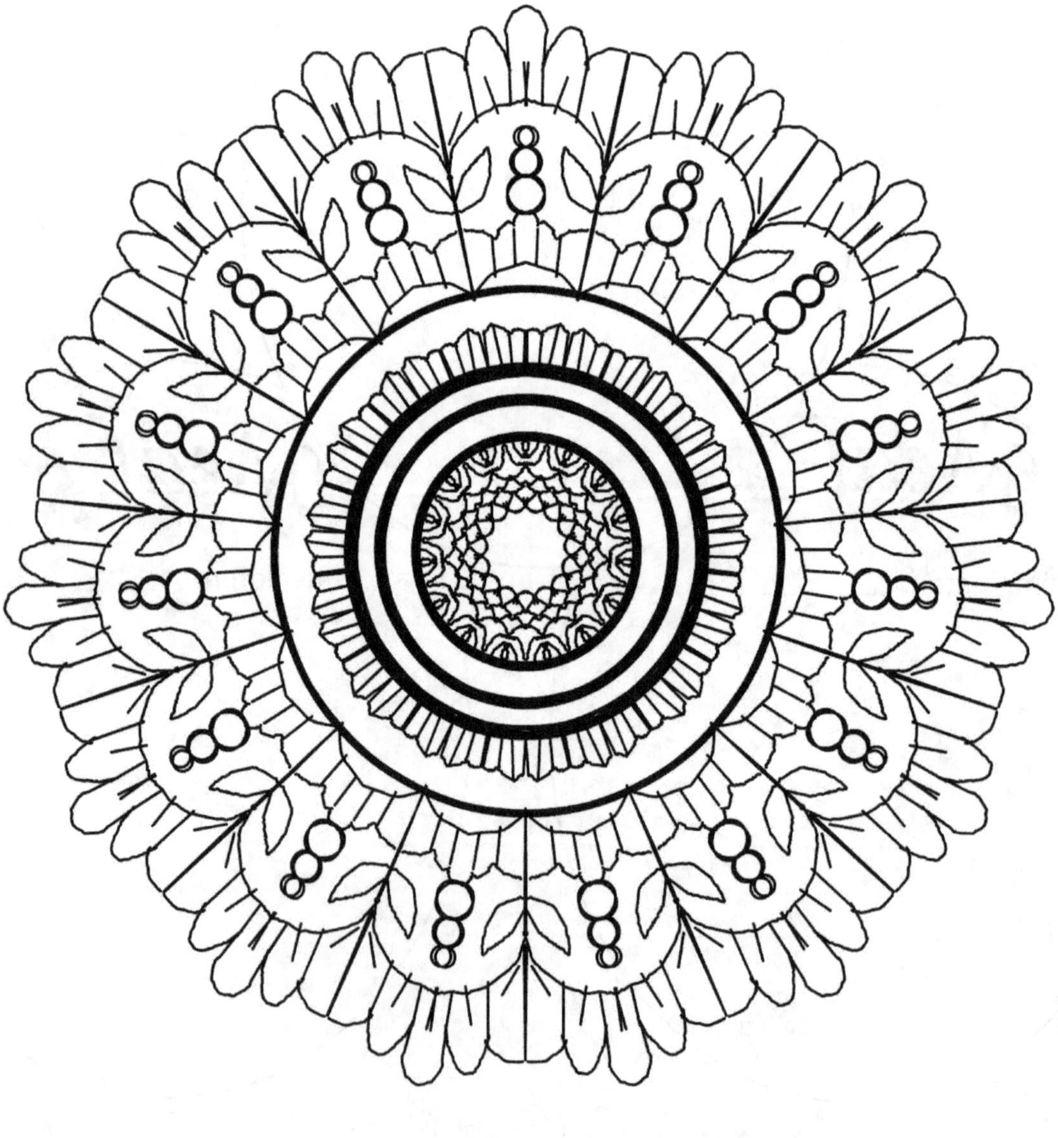

Day Four _______

5:00 _______________________

6:00 _______________________

7:00 _______________________

8:00 _______________________

9:00 _______________________

10:00 _______________________

11:00 _______________________

Noon _______________________

1:00 _______________________

2:00 _______________________

3:00 _______________________

4:00 _______________________

5:00 _______________________

6:00 _______________________

7:00 _______________________

8:00 _______________________

9:00 _______________________

10:00 _______________________

11:00 _______________________

Midnight _______________________

____

____

____

____

Today's victories

What did you commit to today that will make for a better tomorrow?

____

____

____

____

____

____

The Training

Exercise	Set 1	Set 2	Set 3	Set 4	Set 5	notes

Time started: _____________ Time ended: _____________

Location: _______________________________________

Feelings before training:

Feelings aftertraining

NUTRITION

Meal 1

time eaten: _________

Meal 2

time eaten: _________

Meal 3

time eaten: _________

Meal 4

time eaten: _________

Meal 5

time eaten: _________

Hydration

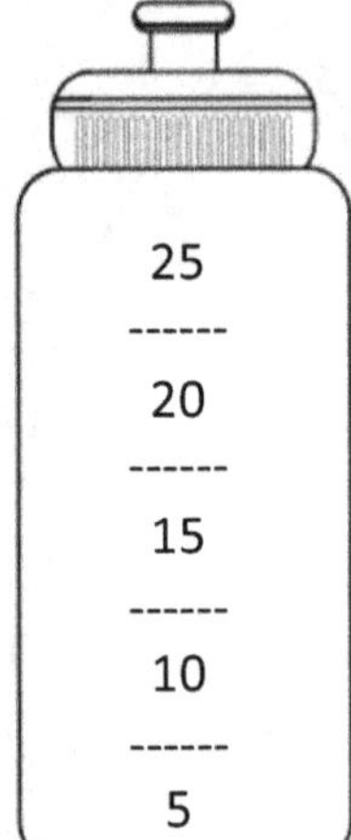

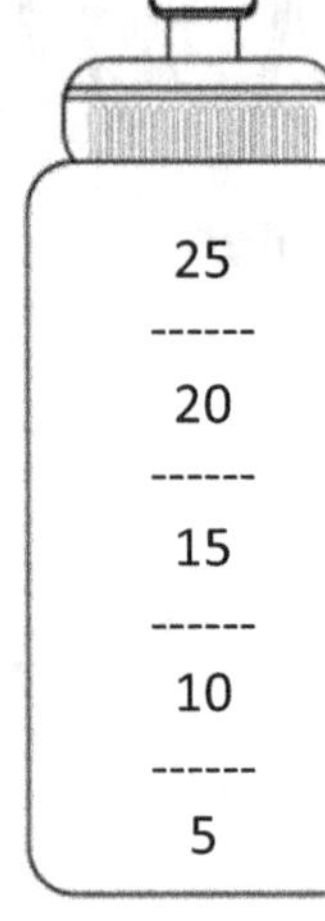

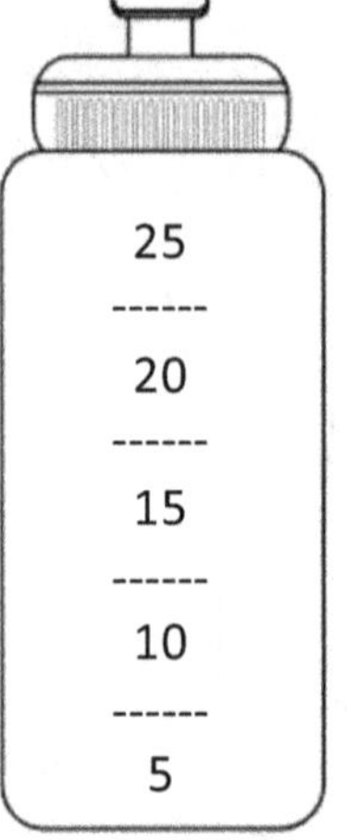

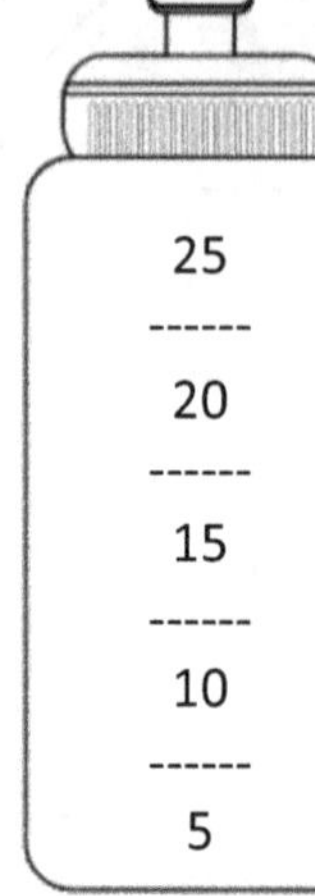

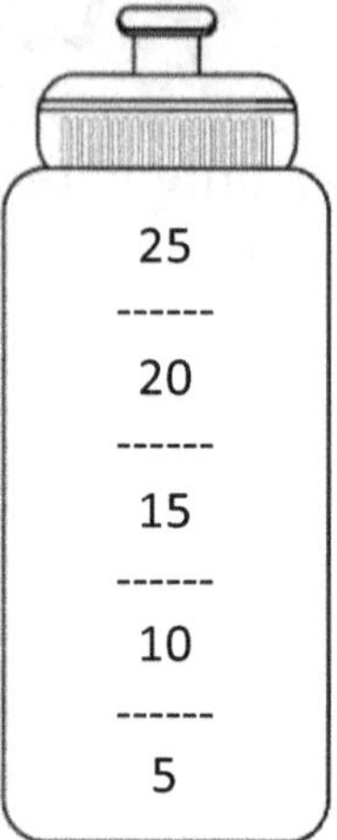

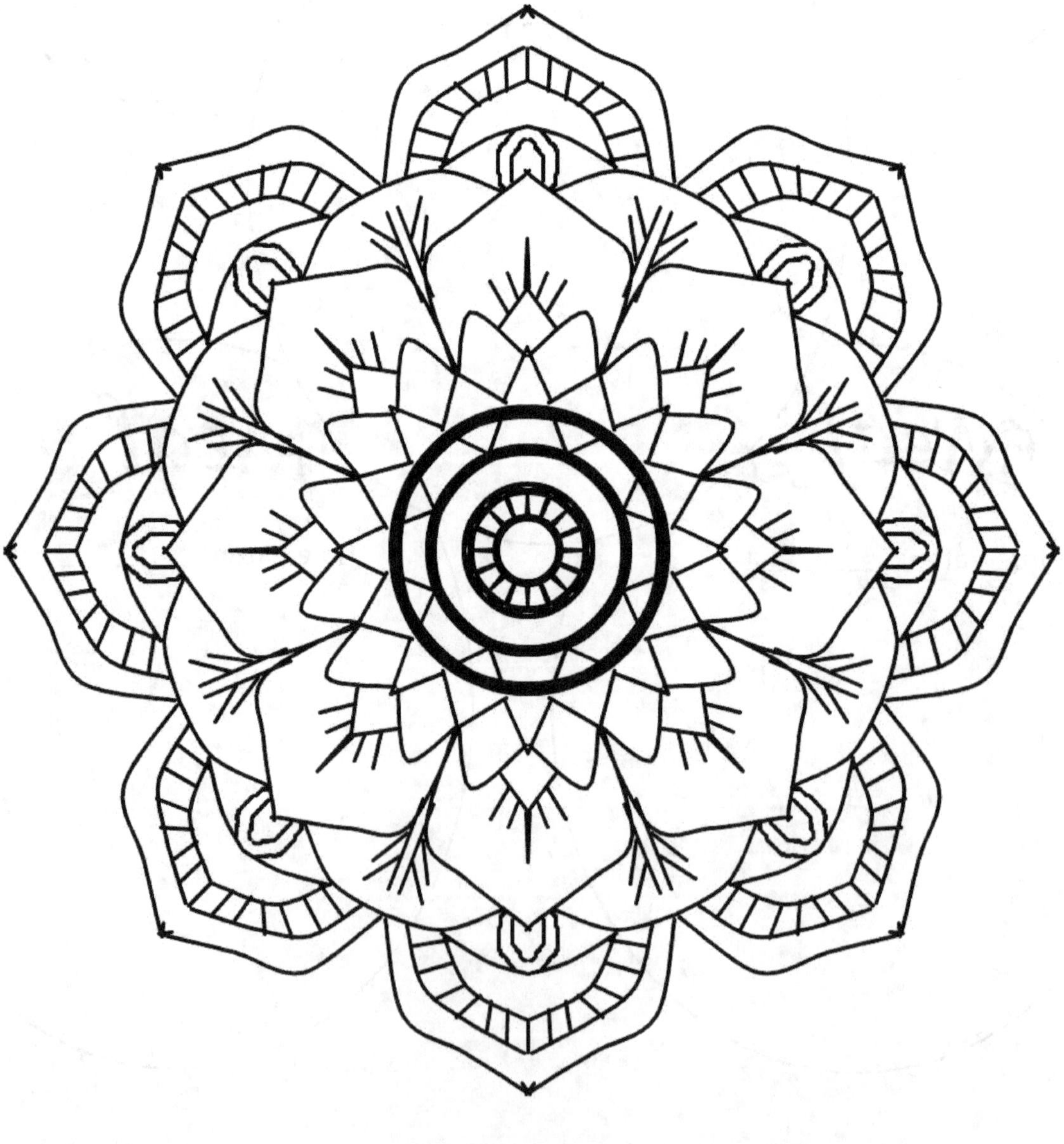

Day Five _______

<table>
<tr><td valign="top">

5:00 ______________________

6:00 ______________________

7:00 ______________________

8:00 ______________________

9:00 ______________________

10:00 _____________________

11:00 _____________________

Noon ______________________

1:00 ______________________

2:00 ______________________

3:00 ______________________

4:00 ______________________

5:00 ______________________

6:00 ______________________

7:00 ______________________

8:00 ______________________

9:00 ______________________

10:00 _____________________

11:00 _____________________

Midnight ___________________

</td><td valign="top">

top priorities for today 🎯

____

____

____

____

____

Today's victories 🏆

Who is the wisest person you know?
Talk to them today.

____

____

____

____

____

____

</td></tr>
</table>

The Training

Exercise	Set 1	Set 2	Set 3	Set 4	Set 5	notes

Time started: _____________ Time ended: _______________

Location: ____

Feelings before training:

Feelings after training

NUTRITION

Meal 1
time eaten: _________

Meal 2
time eaten: _________

Meal 3
time eaten: _________

Meal 4
time eaten: _________

Meal 5
time eaten: _________

Hydration

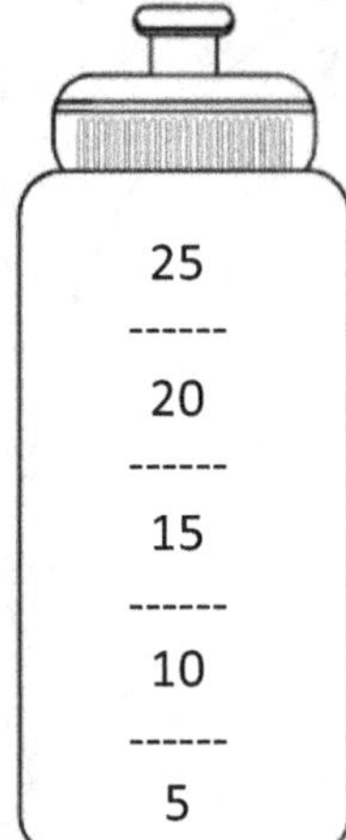
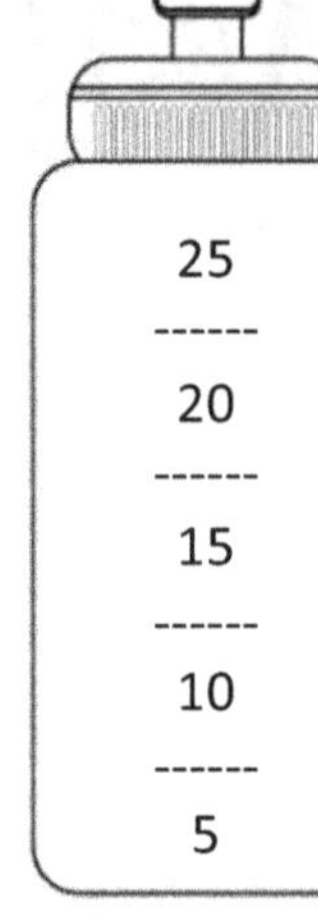
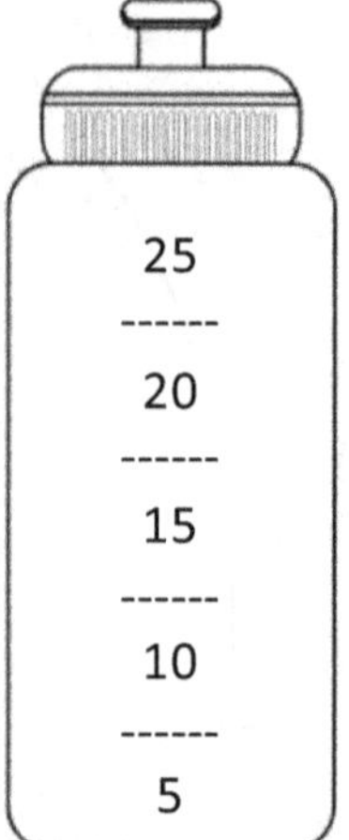
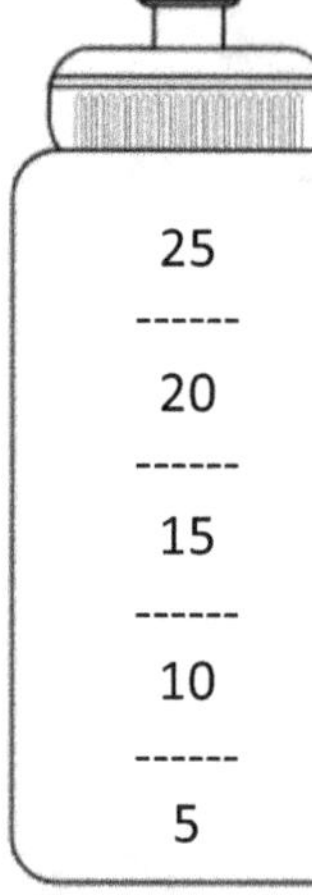
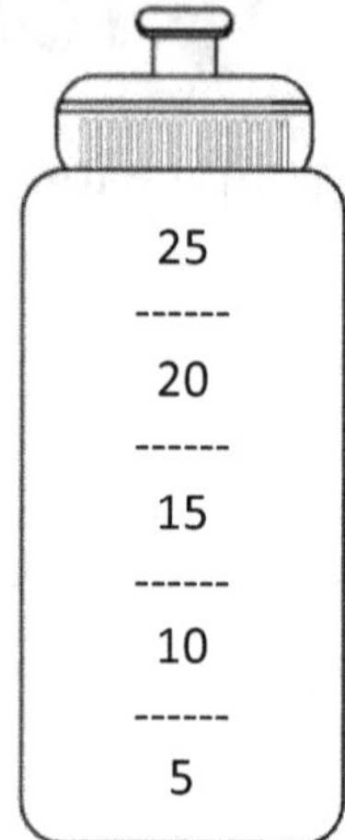

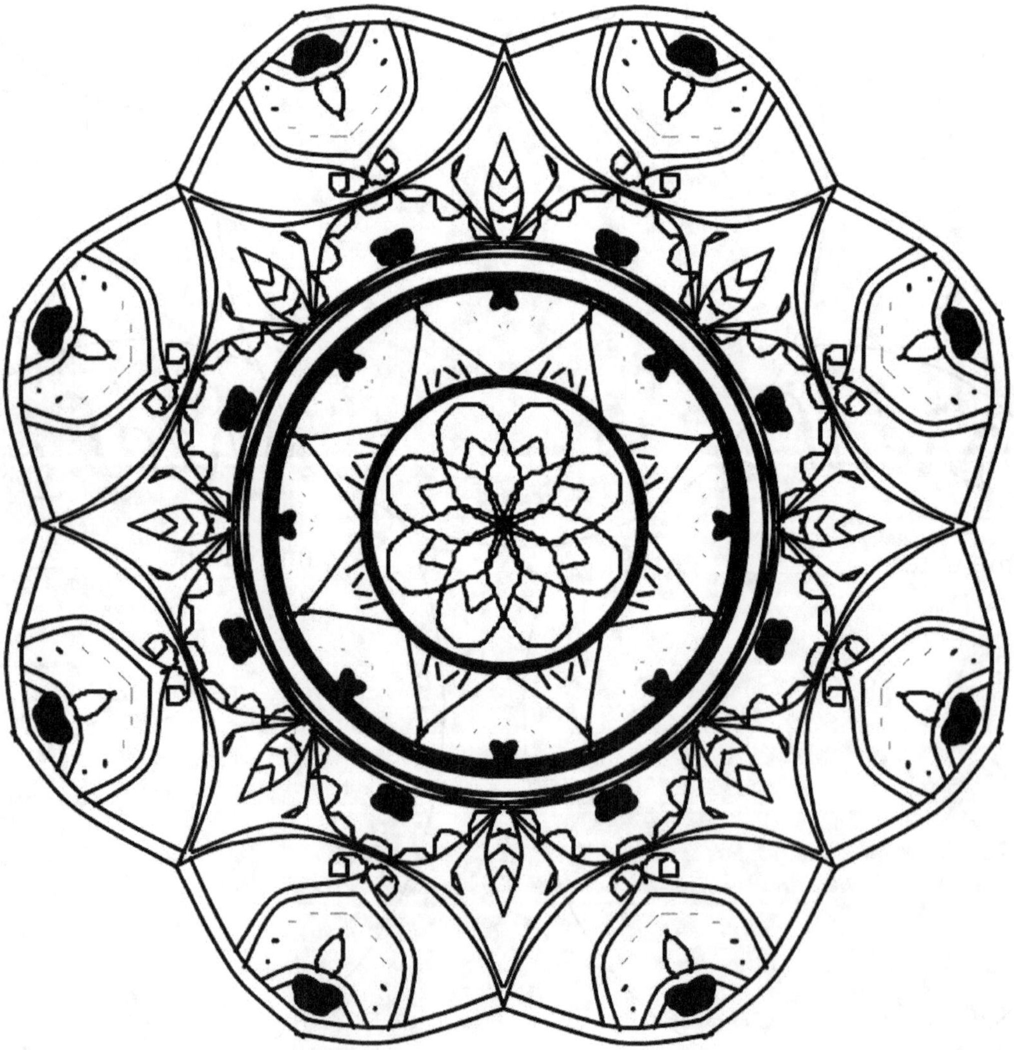

Day Six _______

5:00 ________________	

5:00 _______________________

6:00 _______________________

7:00 _______________________

8:00 _______________________

9:00 _______________________

10:00 ______________________

11:00 ______________________

Noon _______________________

1:00 _______________________

2:00 _______________________

3:00 _______________________

4:00 _______________________

5:00 _______________________

6:00 _______________________

7:00 _______________________

8:00 _______________________

9:00 _______________________

10:00 ______________________

11:00 ______________________

Midnight ___________________

____

____

____

____

____

Today's victories

What is your biggest fear and how do you get over it?

____

____

____

____

____

____

The Training

Exercise	Set 1	Set 2	Set 3	Set 4	Set 5	notes

Time started: _____________ Time ended: _____________

Location: ____

Feelings before training:

Feelings after training

NUTRITION

Meal 1

time eaten: _________

Meal 2

time eaten: _________

Meal 3

time eaten: _________

Meal 4

time eaten: _________

Meal 5

time eaten: _________

Hydration

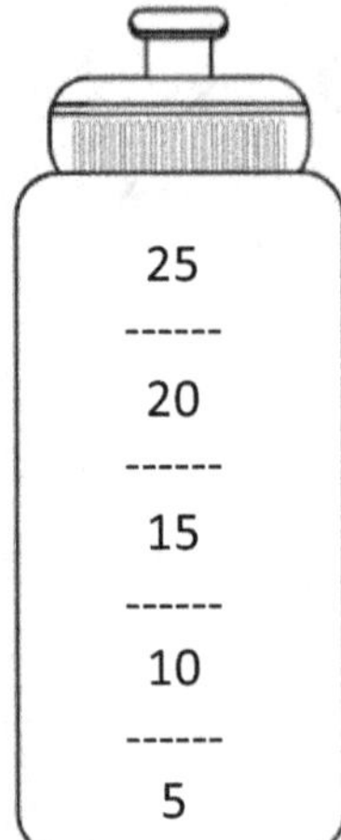

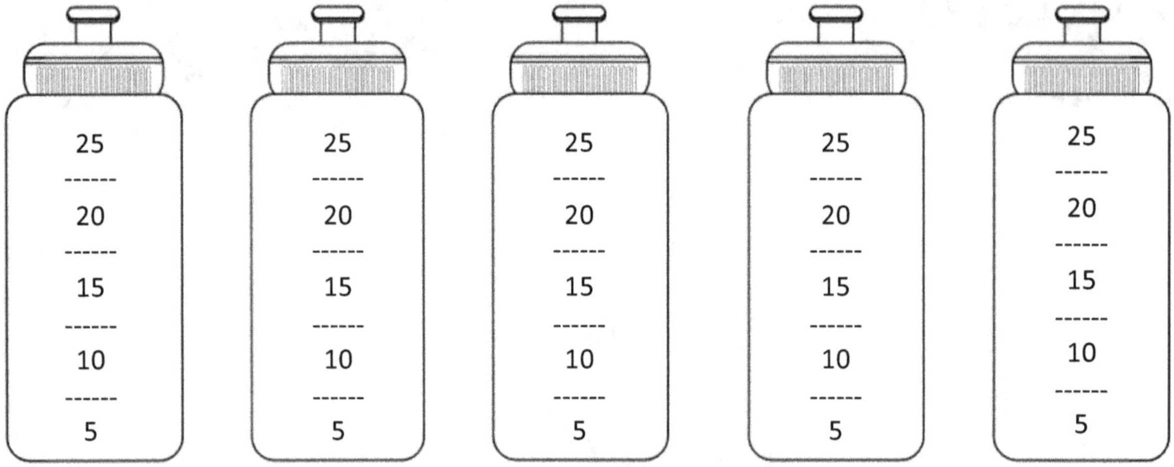

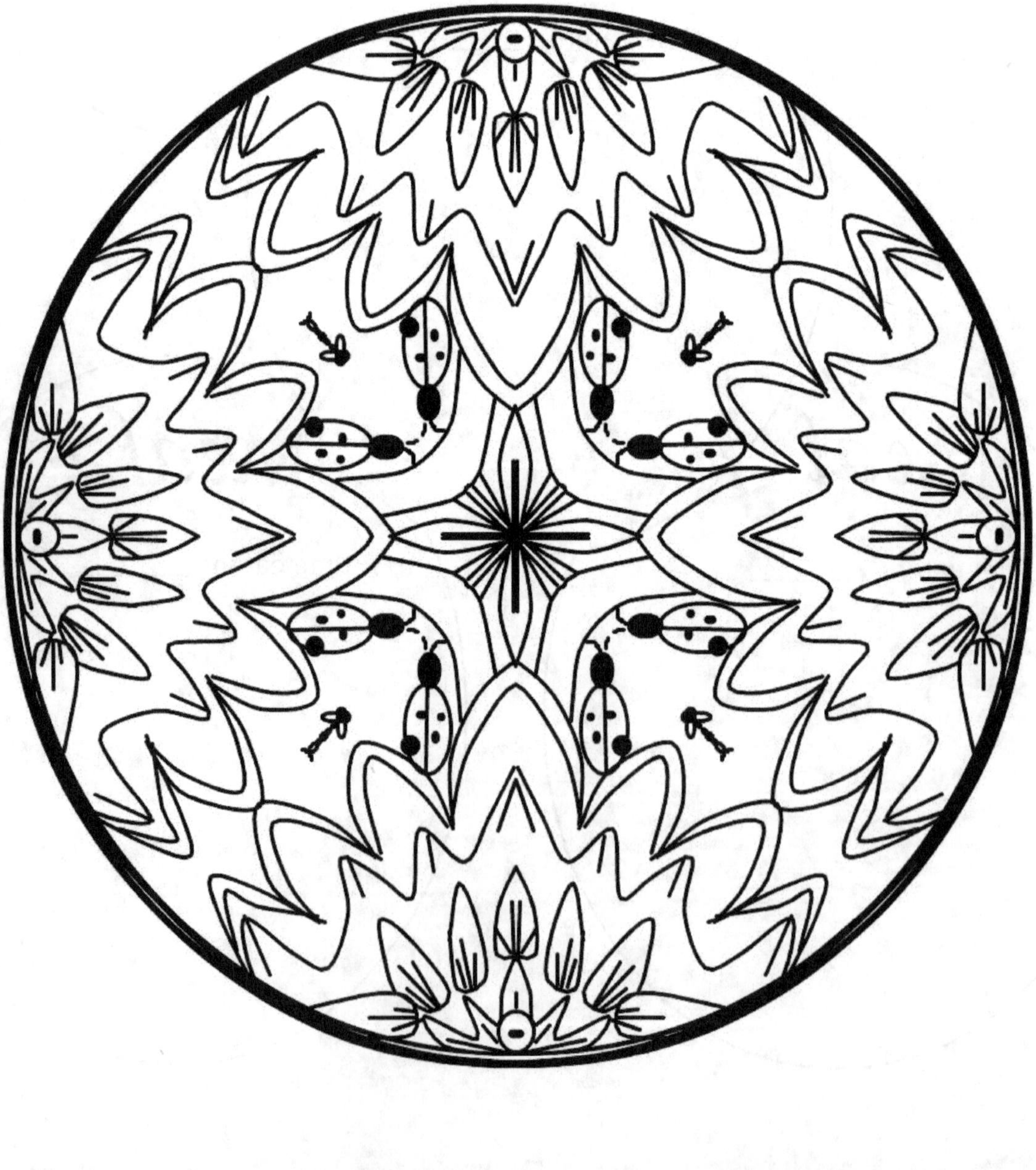

Day Seven _______

5:00 _______________	

5:00 _______________

6:00 _______________

7:00 _______________

8:00 _______________

9:00 _______________

10:00 _______________

11:00 _______________

Noon _______________

1:00 _______________

2:00 _______________

3:00 _______________

4:00 _______________

5:00 _______________

6:00 _______________

7:00 _______________

8:00 _______________

9:00 _______________

10:00 _______________

11:00 _______________

Midnight _______________

top priorities for today

____

____

____

____

Today's victories

Where does your strength
come from?

____

____

____

____

____

____

The *Stella Society* Training

Exercise	Set 1	Set 2	Set 3	Set 4	Set 5	notes

Time started: _____________ Time ended: _____________

Location: ____

Feelings before training: 🙂 😐 ☹️ 😜 😠 😕 😇 😎

Feelings after training 🙂 😐 ☹️ 😜 😠 😕 😇 😎

NUTRITION

Meal 1
time eaten: _________

Meal 2
time eaten: _________

Meal 3
time eaten: _________

Meal 4
time eaten: _________

Meal 5
time eaten: _________

Hydration

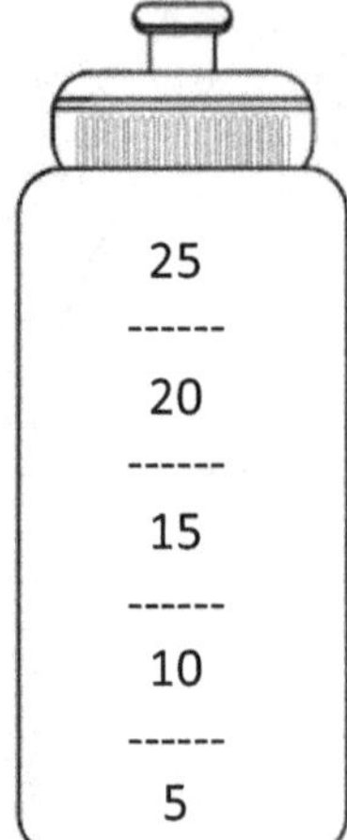

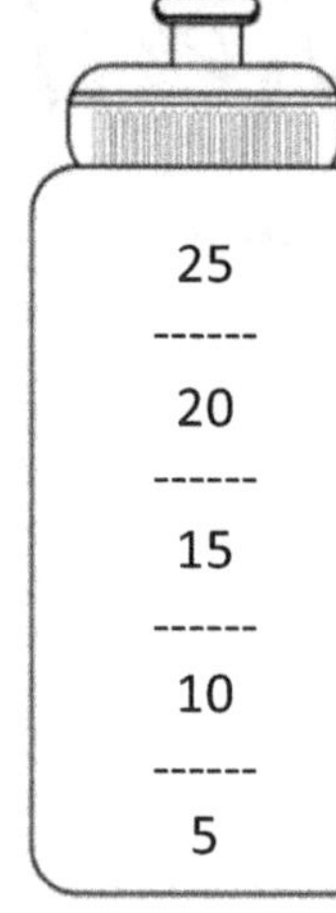

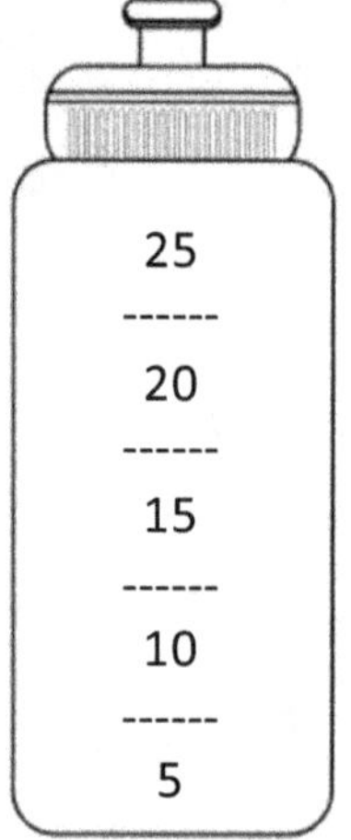

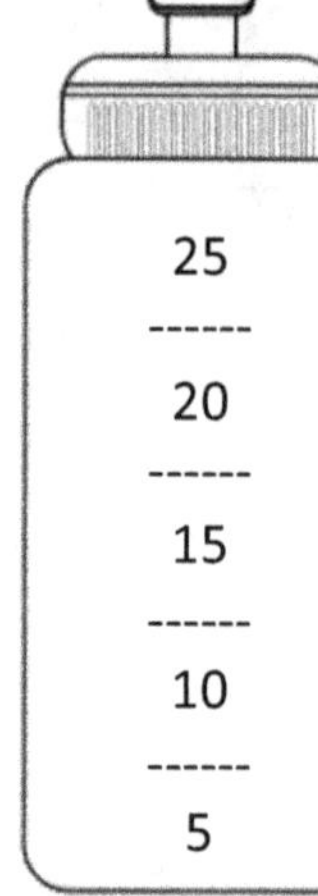

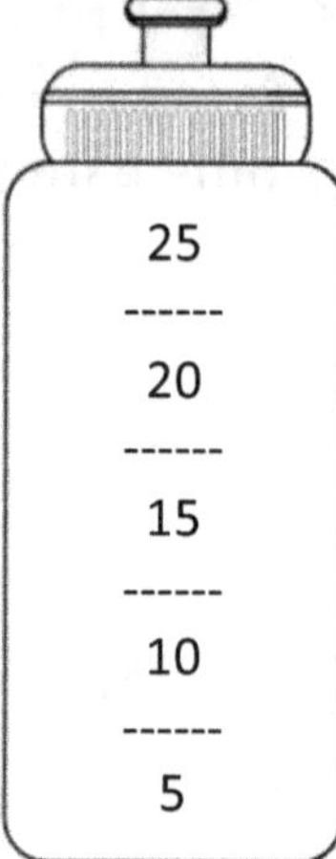

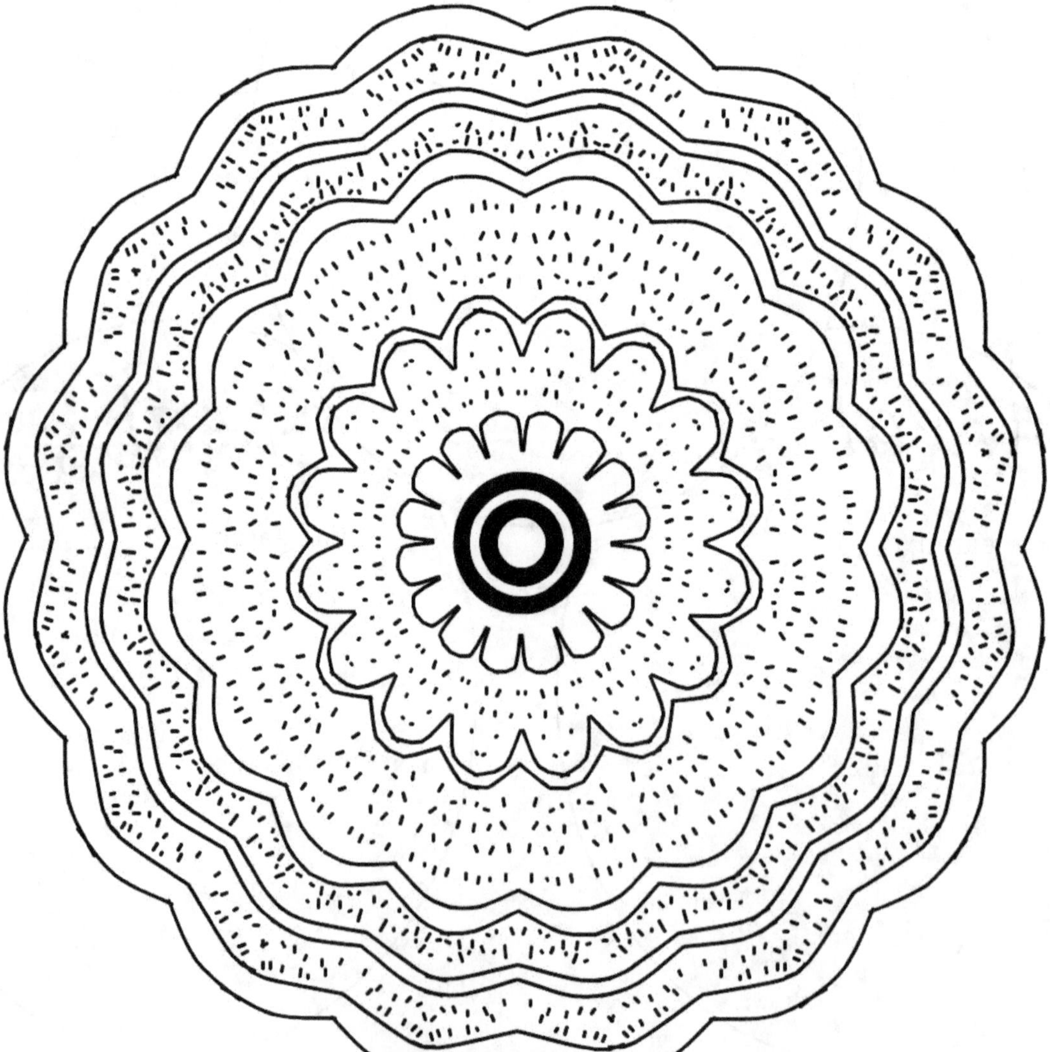

Day Eight _______

5:00 _______________________

6:00 _______________________

7:00 _______________________

8:00 _______________________

9:00 _______________________

10:00 ______________________

11:00 ______________________

Noon _______________________

1:00 _______________________

2:00 _______________________

3:00 _______________________

4:00 _______________________

5:00 _______________________

6:00 _______________________

7:00 _______________________

8:00 _______________________

9:00 _______________________

10:00 ______________________

11:00 ______________________

Midnight ___________________

top priorities for today 🎯

____

____

____

____

Today's victories 🏆

What motivates you to be
the best version of you?

____

____

____

____

____

____

The Training

Exercise	Set 1	Set 2	Set 3	Set 4	Set 5	notes

Time started: _____________ Time ended: _____________

Location: _______________________________________

Feelings before training:

Feelings after training

NUTRITION

Meal 1

time eaten: _________

Meal 2

time eaten: _________

Meal 3

time eaten: _________

Meal 4

time eaten: _________

Meal 5

time eaten: _________

Hydration

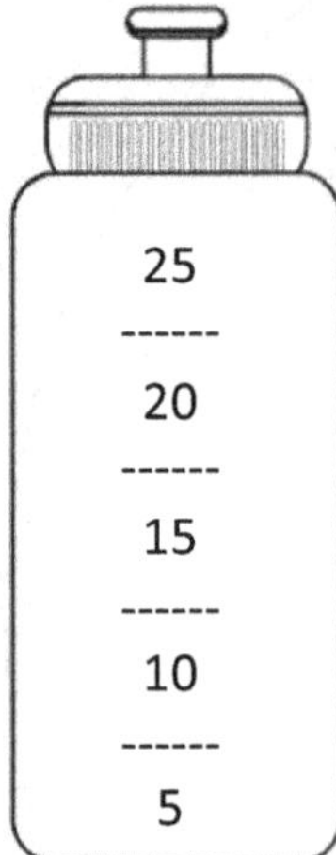

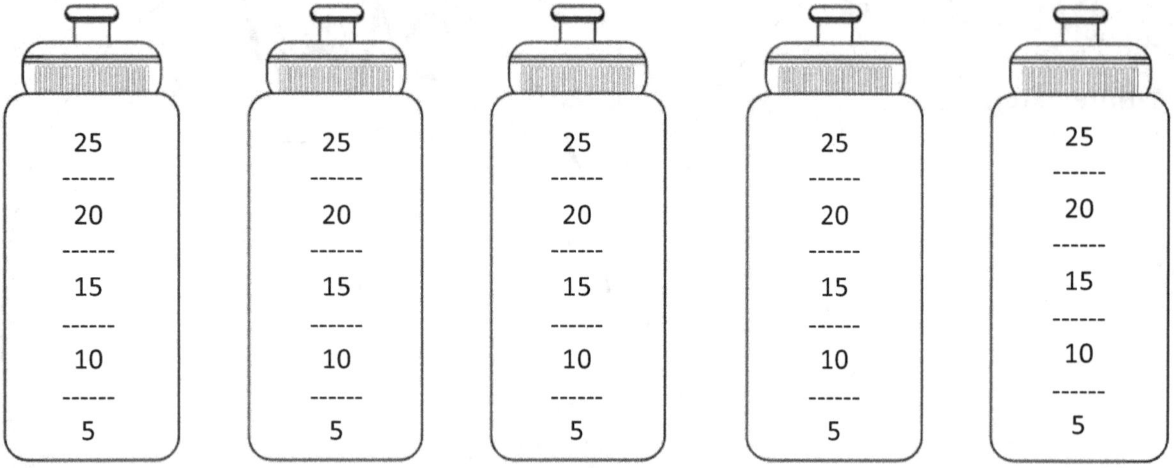

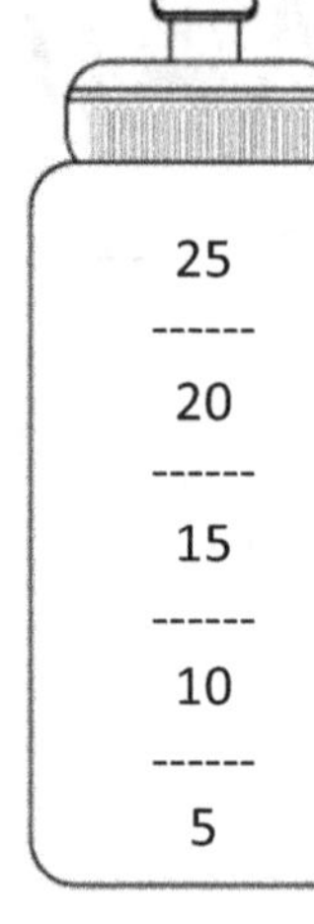

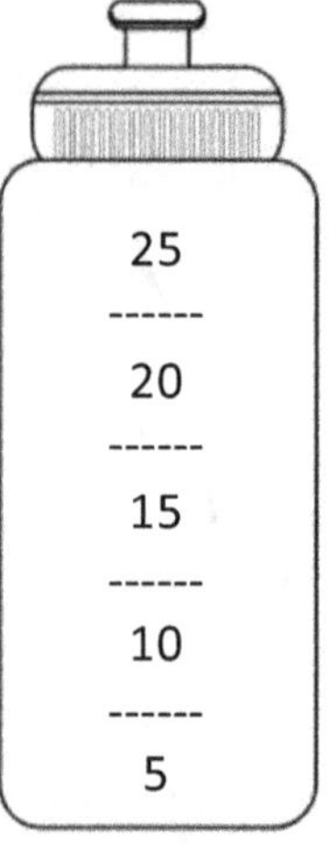

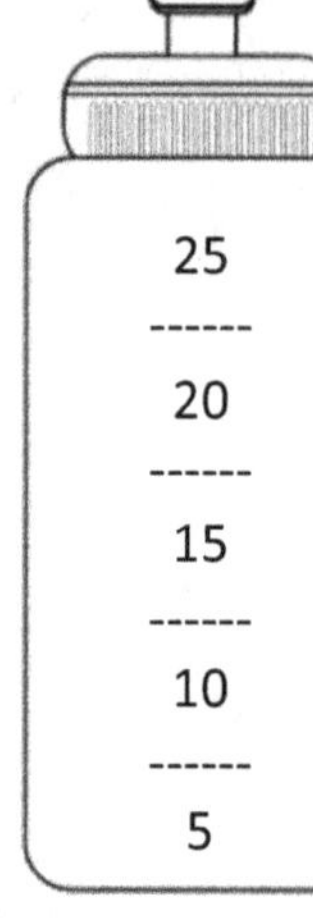

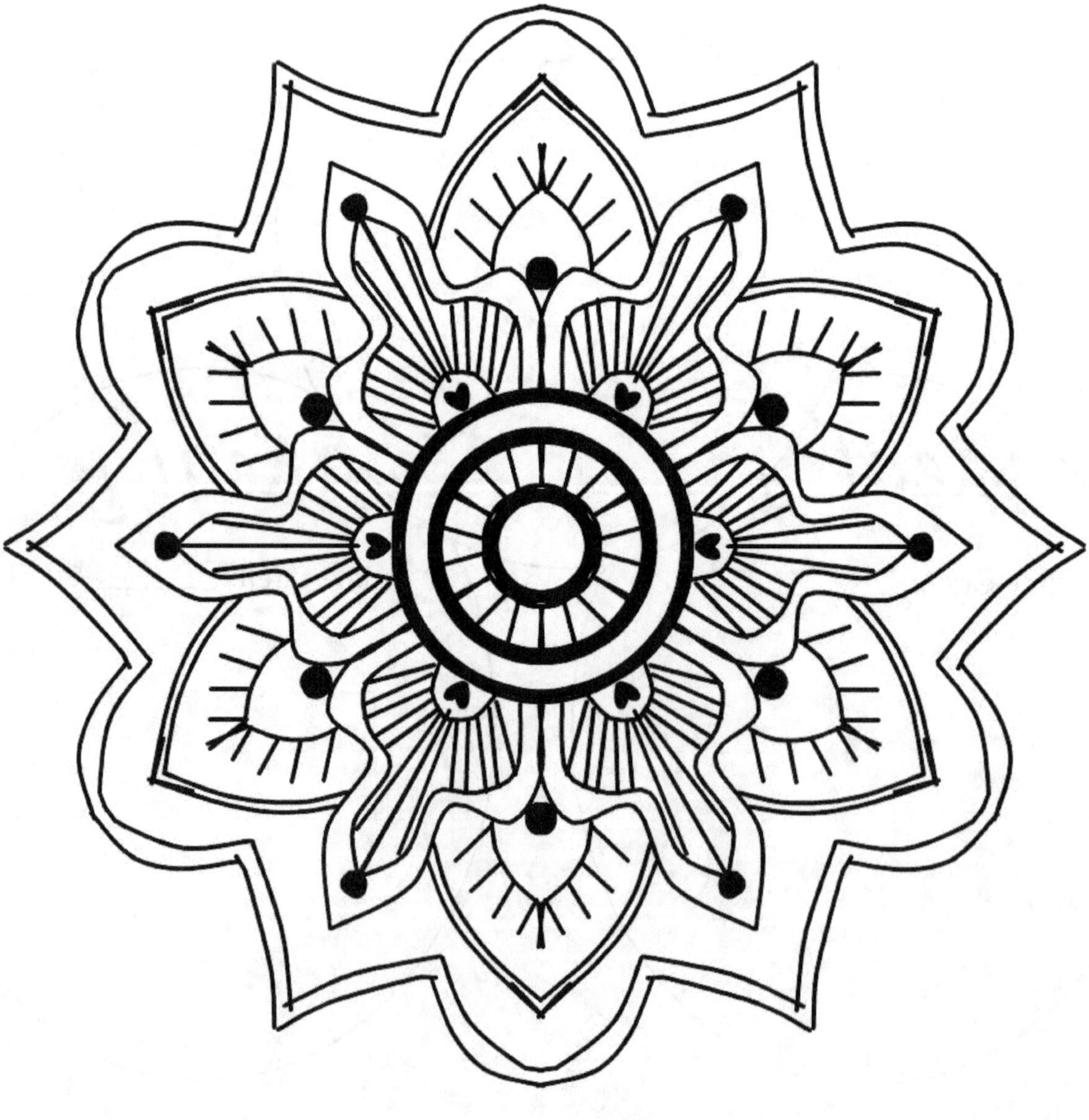

Day Nine _______

5:00 _______________________

6:00 _______________________

7:00 _______________________

8:00 _______________________

9:00 _______________________

10:00 ______________________

11:00 ______________________

Noon _______________________

1:00 _______________________

2:00 _______________________

3:00 _______________________

4:00 _______________________

5:00 _______________________

6:00 _______________________

7:00 _______________________

8:00 _______________________

9:00 _______________________

10:00 ______________________

11:00 ______________________

Midnight ____________________

top priorities for today 🎯

____

____

____

____

____

Today's victories 🏆

How will you be consistent
this week?

____

____

____

____

____

____

The *Stella Society* Training

Exercise	Set 1	Set 2	Set 3	Set 4	Set 5	notes

Time started: _______________   Time ended: _______________

Location: ____

Feelings before training: 🙂 😐 🙁 😜 😣 😟 😊 😎

Feelings after training 🙂 😐 🙁 😜 😣 😟 😊 😎

NUTRITION

Meal 1

time eaten: _________

Meal 2

time eaten: _________

Meal 3

time eaten: _________

Meal 4

time eaten: _________

Meal 5

time eaten: _________

Hydration

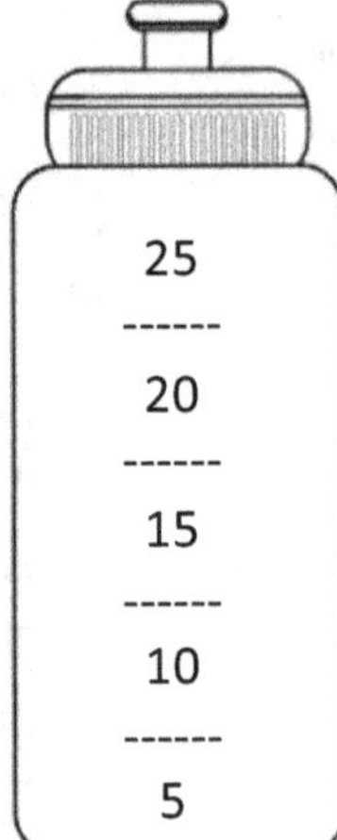

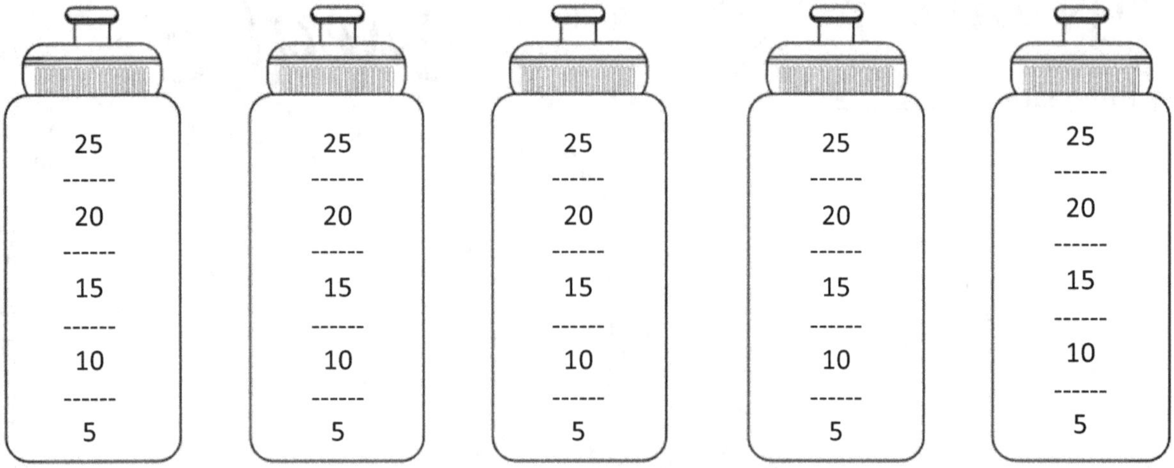

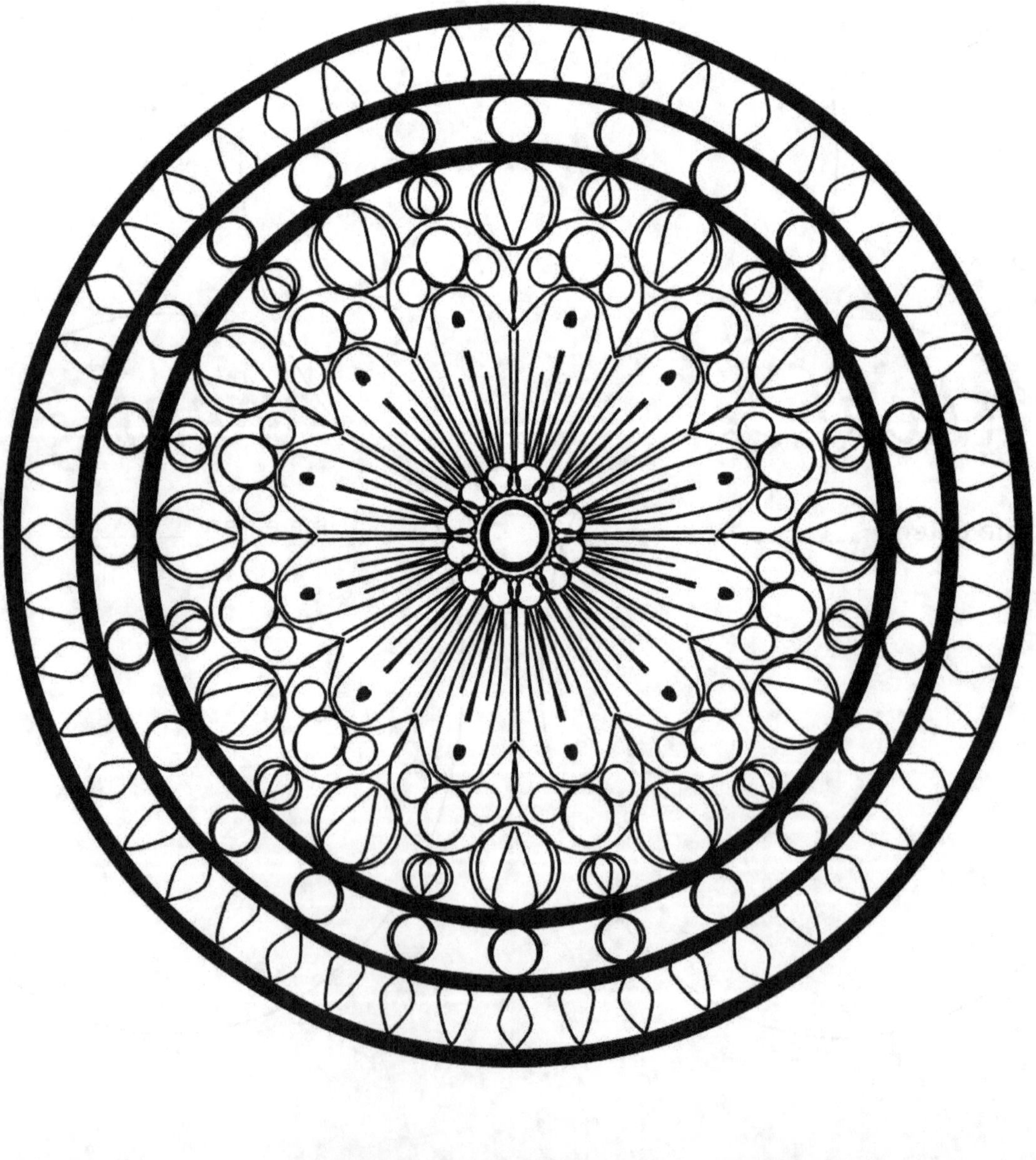

Day Ten _______

5:00 _______________________

6:00 _______________________

7:00 _______________________

8:00 _______________________

9:00 _______________________

10:00 ______________________

11:00 ______________________

Noon _______________________

1:00 _______________________

2:00 _______________________

3:00 _______________________

4:00 _______________________

5:00 _______________________

6:00 _______________________

7:00 _______________________

8:00 _______________________

9:00 _______________________

10:00 ______________________

11:00 ______________________

Midnight ___________________

top priorities for today 🎯

____

____

____

____

Today's victories 🏆

List 5 ways you are loving.

____

____

____

____

____

____

The Training

Exercise	Set 1	Set 2	Set 3	Set 4	Set 5	notes

Time started: _____________ Time ended: _____________

Location: ____

Feelings before training:

Feelings after training

NUTRITION

Meal 1
time eaten: __________

Meal 2
time eaten: __________

Meal 3
time eaten: __________

Meal 4
time eaten: __________

Meal 5
time eaten: __________

Hydration

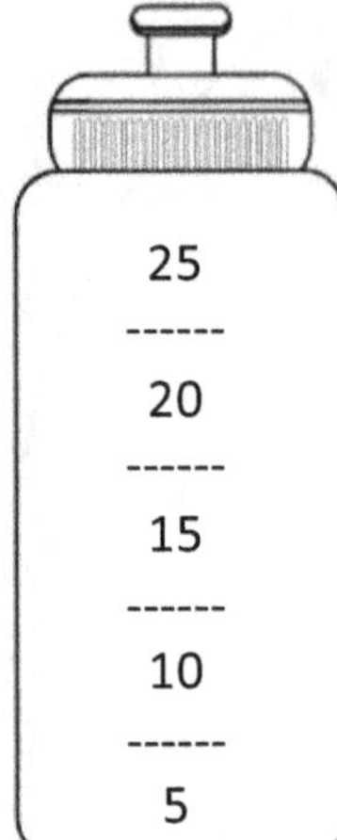

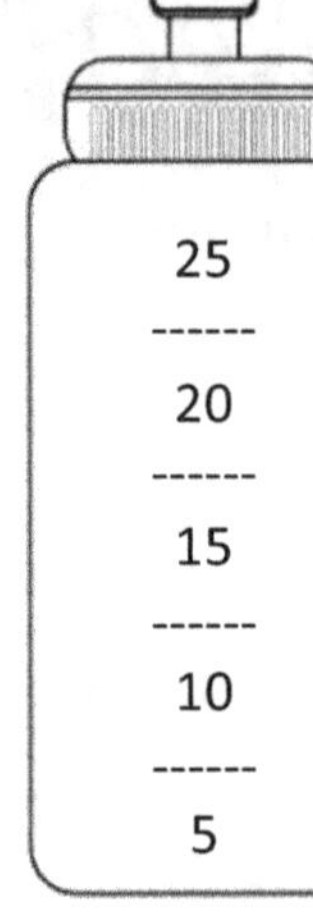

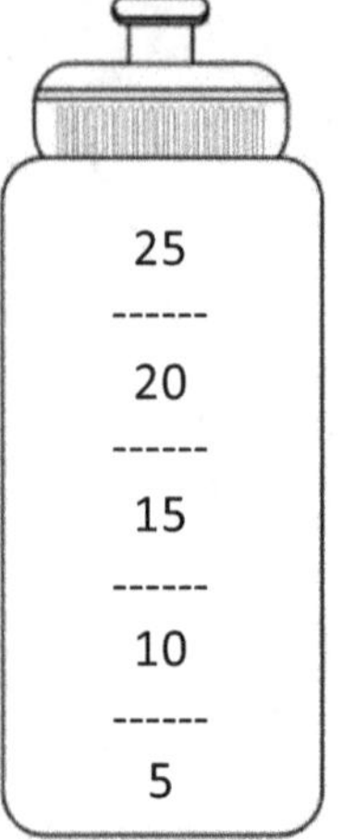

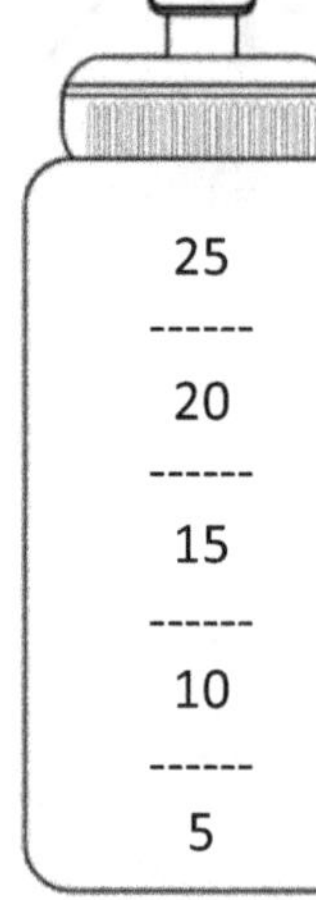

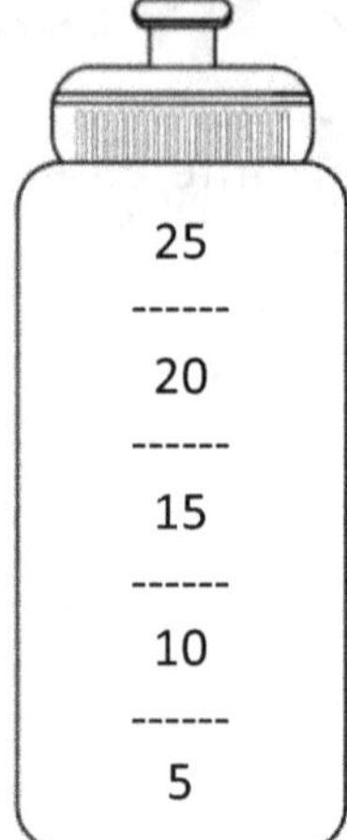

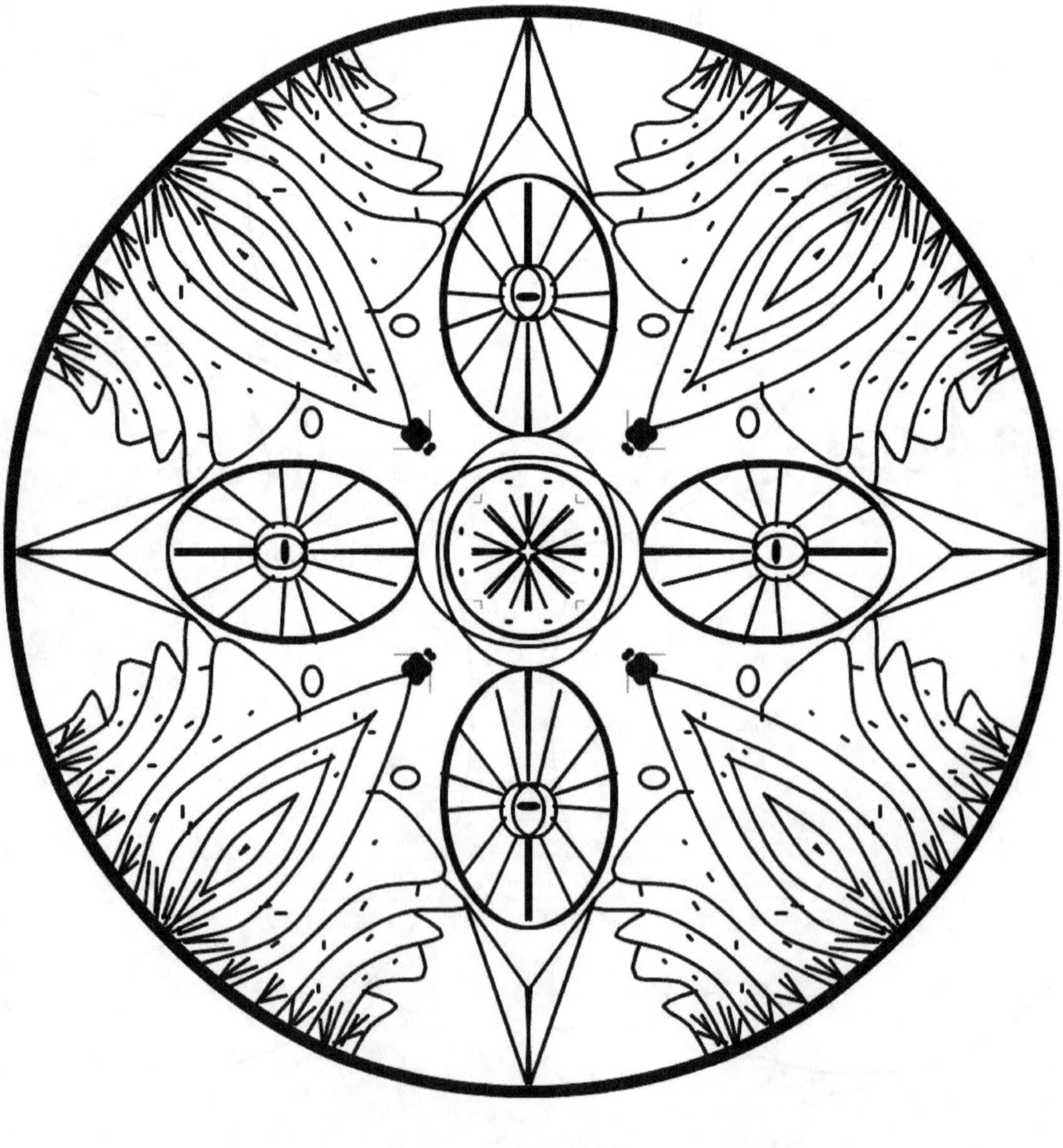

Measurements

DATE: ___________

Weight: _______

Neck _______

Shoulders _______

Chest _______

Bicep / upper arm left _________ right _______

Forearm left _________ right _______

Waist _______

Hips _______

Thighs left _________ right _____

Calf left _________ right _______

The Struggle You Are In Today, Is Developing The Strength You Need for Tomorrow.

Day Eleven _______

5:00 _______________	

5:00 ______________________

6:00 ______________________

7:00 ______________________

8:00 ______________________

9:00 ______________________

10:00 _____________________

11:00 _____________________

Noon _____________________

1:00 ______________________

2:00 ______________________

3:00 ______________________

4:00 ______________________

5:00 ______________________

6:00 ______________________

7:00 ______________________

8:00 ______________________

9:00 ______________________

10:00 _____________________

11:00 _____________________

Midnight ________________

top priorities for today 🎯

____

____

____

____

Today's victories 🏆

Give out as many hugs as you can today. How many did you give?

____

____

____

____

____

The Stella Society Training

Exercise	Set 1	Set 2	Set 3	Set 4	Set 5	notes

Time started: _______________ Time ended: _______________

Location: ____

Feelings before training: 🙂 😐 🙁 😜 😣 😟 😊 😎

Feelings after training 🙂 😐 🙁 😜 😣 😟 😊 😎

NUTRITION

Meal 1
time eaten: _________

Meal 2
time eaten: _________

Meal 3
time eaten: _________

Meal 4
time eaten: _________

Meal 5
time eaten: _________

Hydration

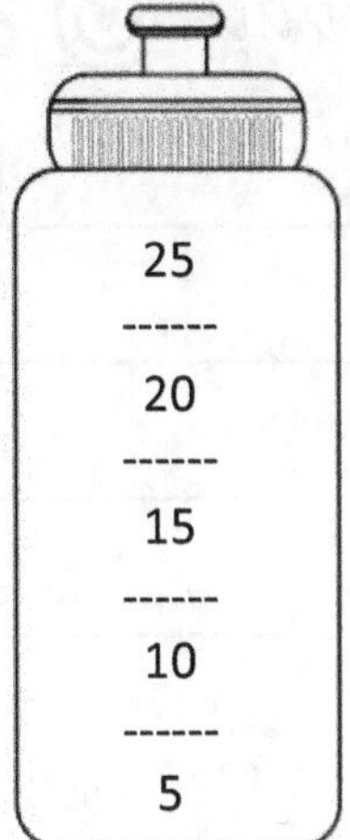

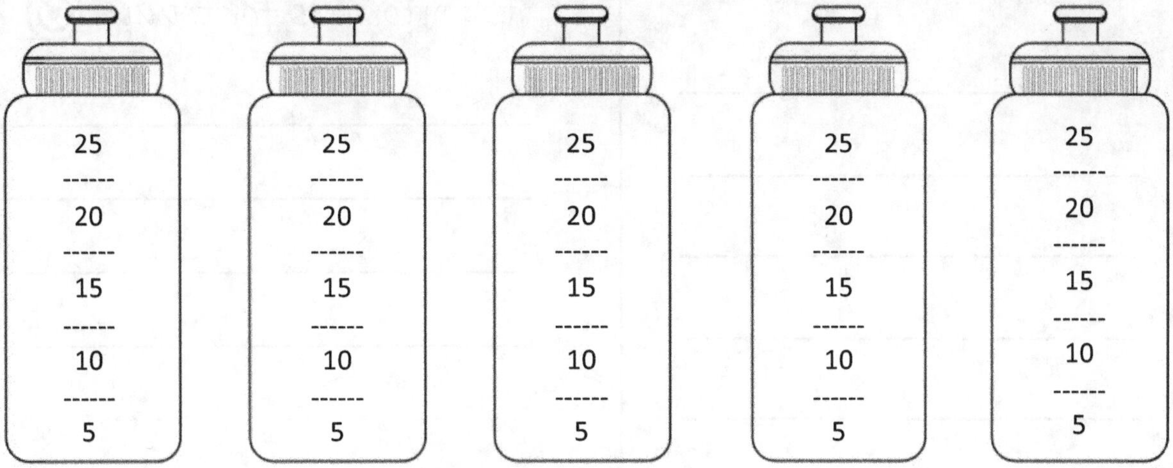

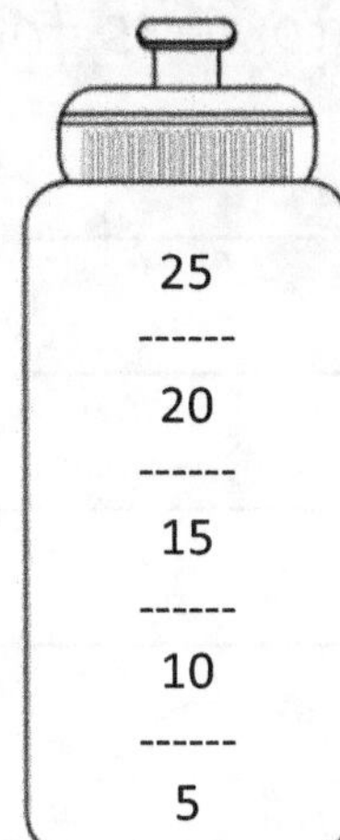

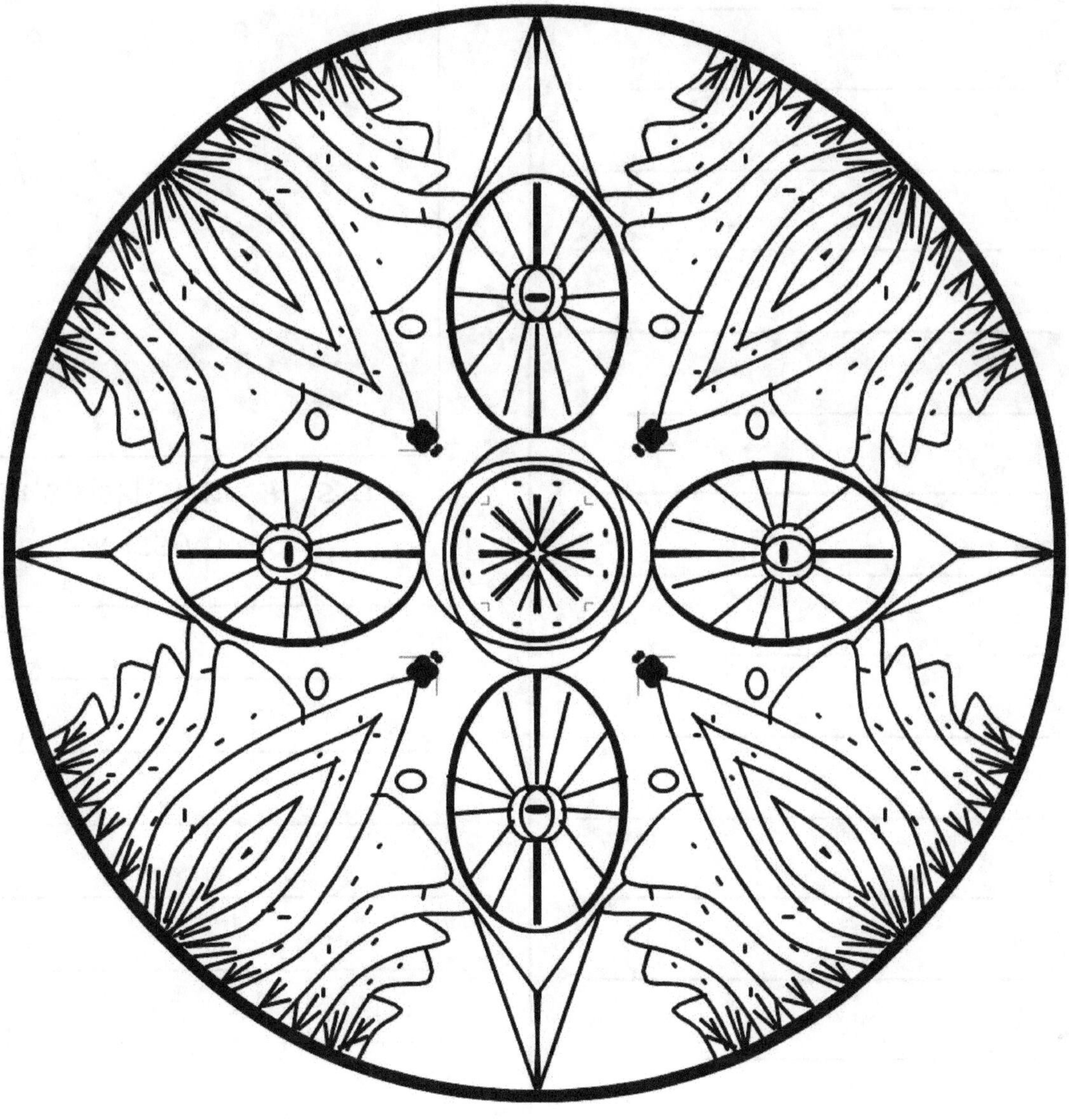

Day Twelve _______

 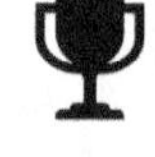

5:00 ______________________

6:00 ______________________

7:00 ______________________

8:00 ______________________

9:00 ______________________

10:00 _____________________

11:00 _____________________

Noon _____________________

1:00 ______________________

2:00 ______________________

3:00 ______________________

4:00 ______________________

5:00 ______________________

6:00 ______________________

7:00 ______________________

8:00 ______________________

9:00 ______________________

10:00 _____________________

11:00 _____________________

Midnight ________________

____

____

____

____

Today's victories 🏆

List 4 ways you show compassion.

____

____

____

____

____

The *Stella Society* Training

Exercise	Set 1	Set 2	Set 3	Set 4	Set 5	notes

Time started: _____________ Time ended: _____________

Location: ____

Feelings before training: 🙂 😐 🙁 😜 😠 😟 😊 😎

Feelings after training 🙂 😐 🙁 😜 😠 😟 😊 😎

NUTRITION

Meal 1

time eaten: _________

Meal 2

time eaten: _________

Meal 3

time eaten: _________

Meal 4

time eaten: _________

Meal 5

time eaten: _________

Hydration

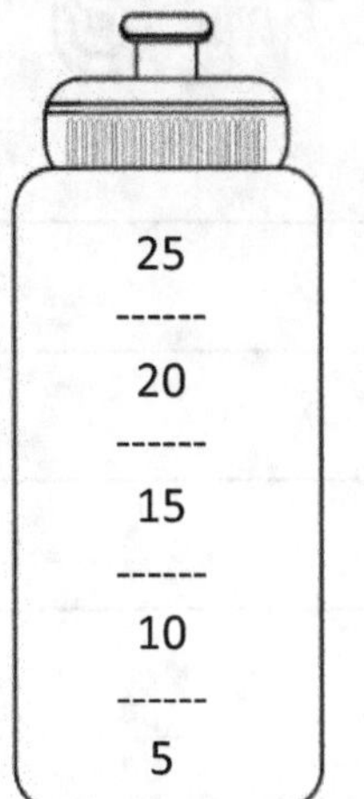

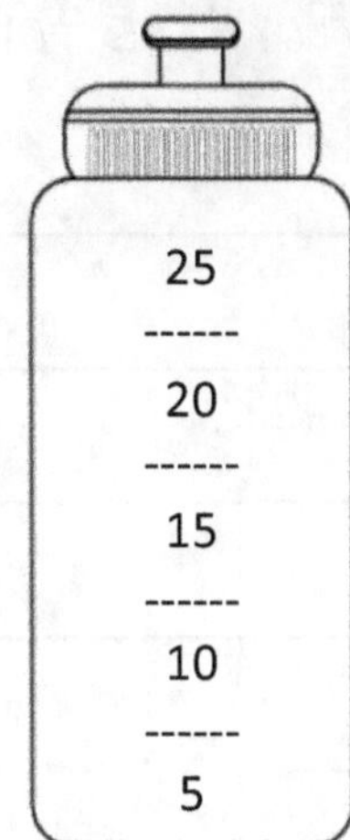

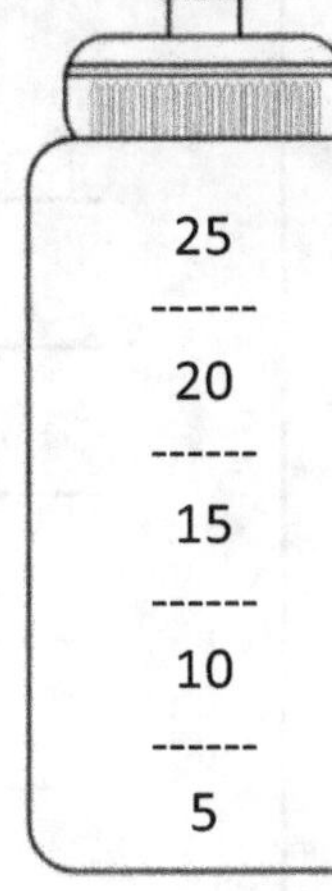

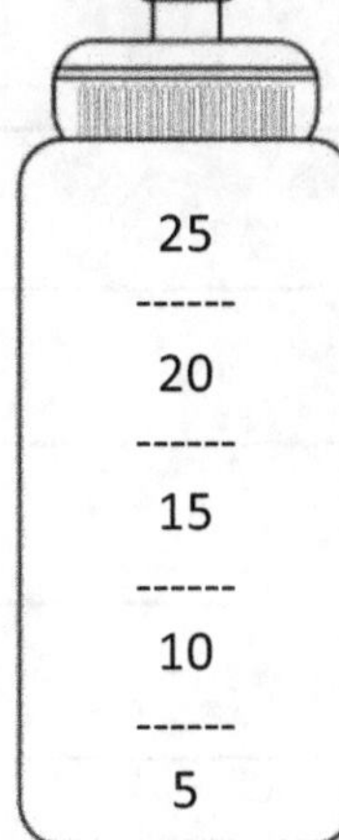

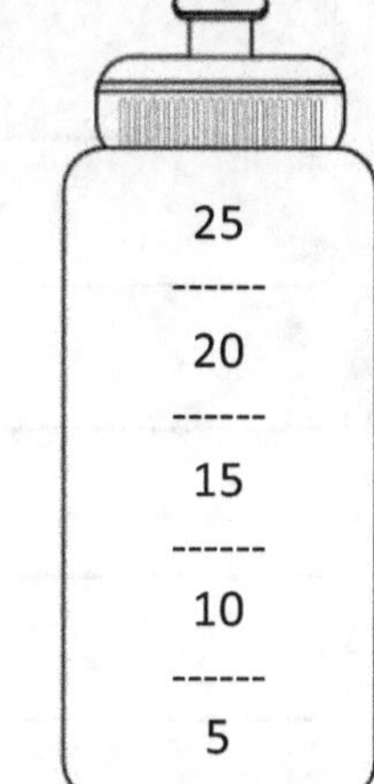

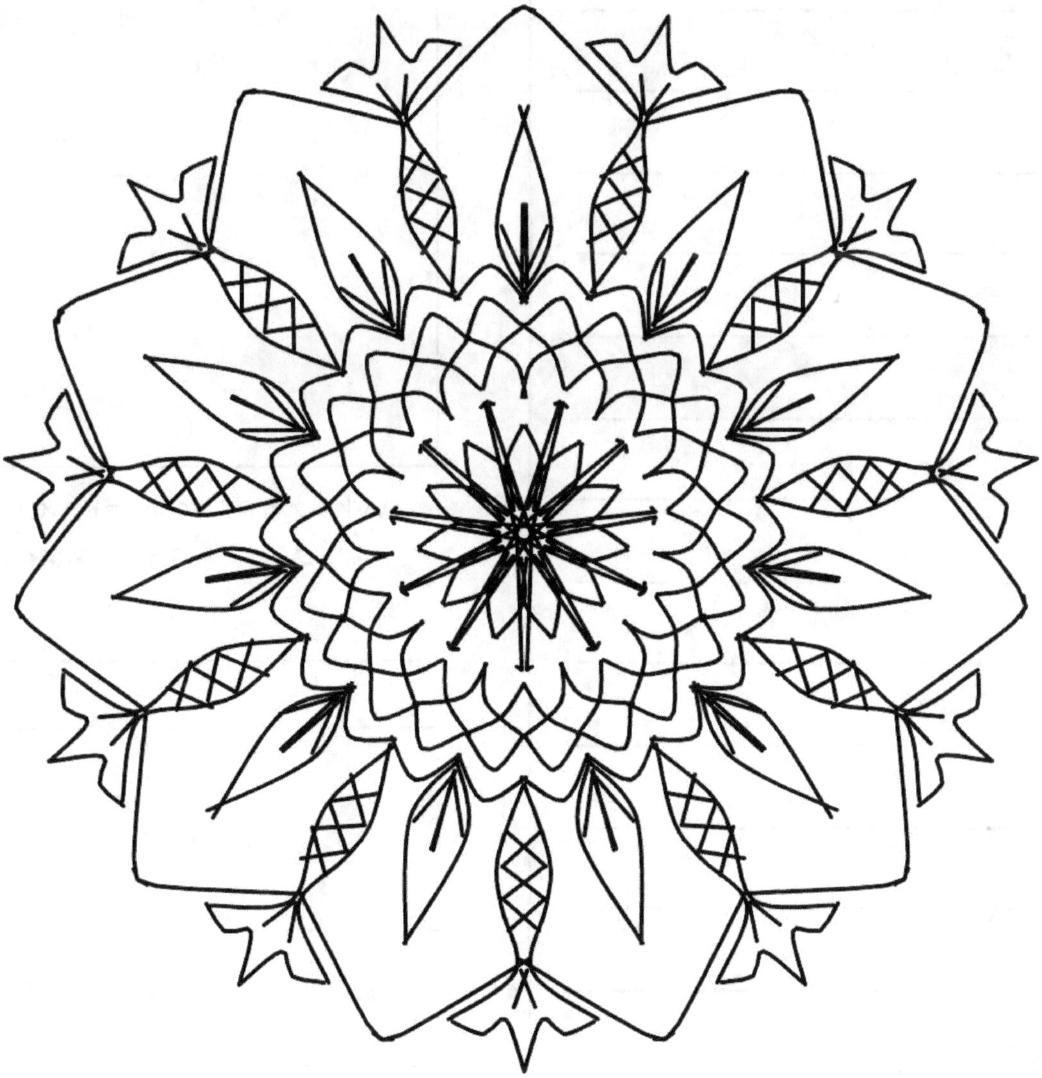

Day Thirteen ______

5:00 ___________________

6:00 ___________________

7:00 ___________________

8:00 ___________________

9:00 ___________________

10:00 ___________________

11:00 ___________________

Noon ___________________

1:00 ___________________

2:00 ___________________

3:00 ___________________

4:00 ___________________

5:00 ___________________

6:00 ___________________

7:00 ___________________

8:00 ___________________

9:00 ___________________

10:00 ___________________

11:00 ___________________

Midnight ___________________

top priorities for today

Today's victories

Who needs roses from your garden and why?

The Stella Society Training

Exercise	Set 1	Set 2	Set 3	Set 4	Set 5	notes

Time started: _______________ Time ended: _______________

Location: ____

Feelings before training:        

Feelings after training

NUTRITION

Meal 1

time eaten: _________

Meal 2

time eaten: _________

Meal 3

time eaten: _________

Meal 4

time eaten: _________

Meal 5

time eaten: _________

Hydration

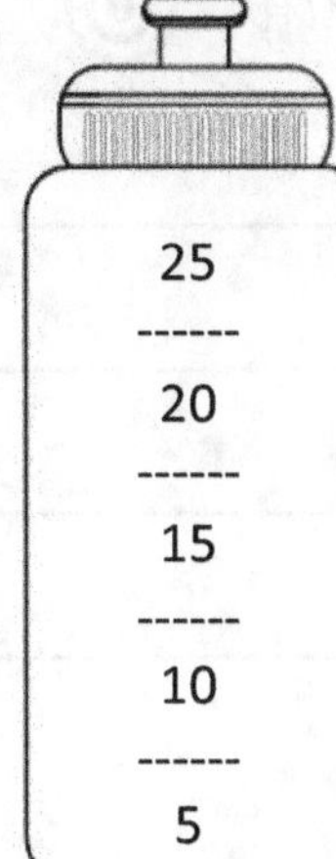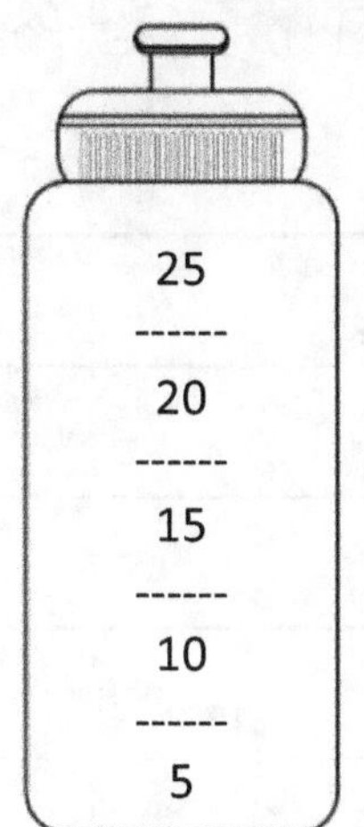

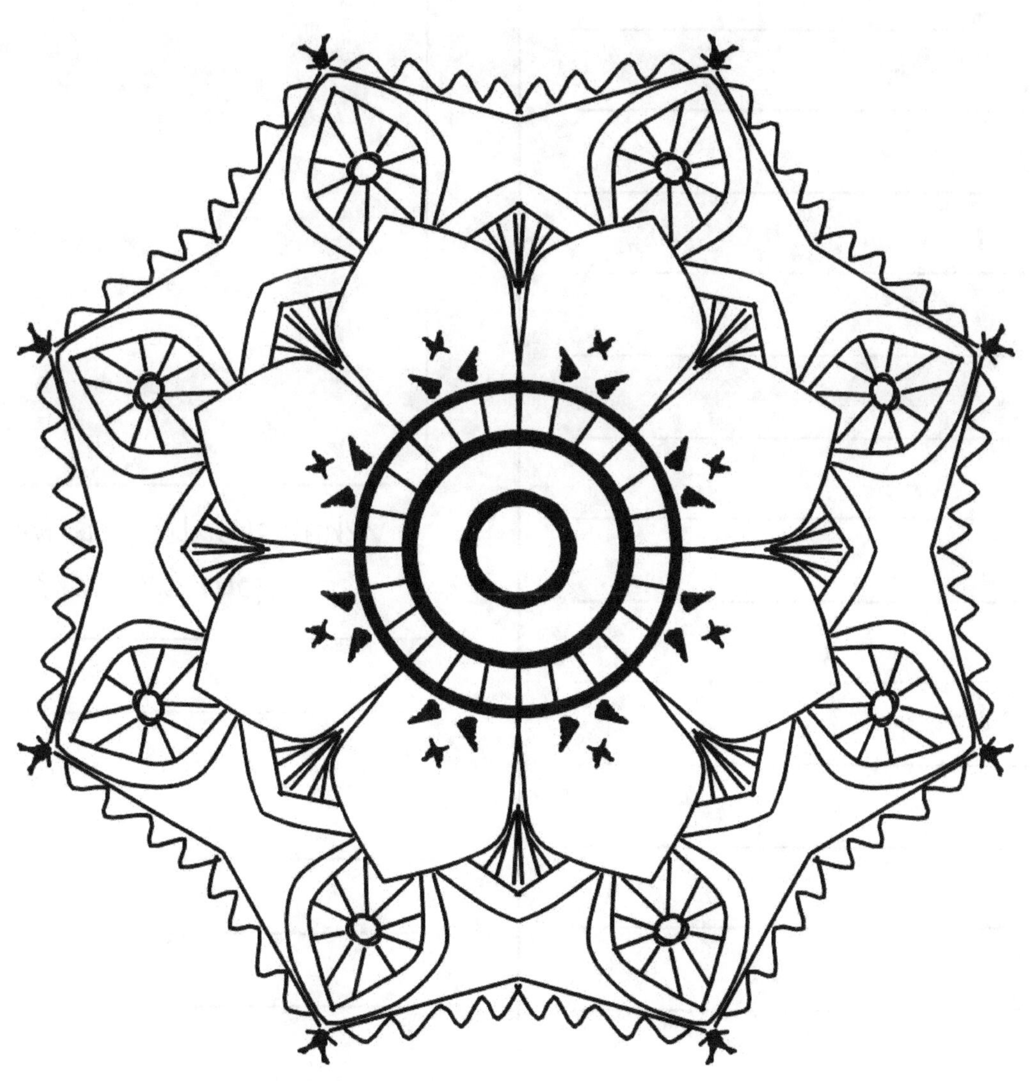

Day Fourteen _______

5:00 _______________________

6:00 _______________________

7:00 _______________________

8:00 _______________________

9:00 _______________________

10:00 ______________________

11:00 ______________________

Noon _______________________

1:00 _______________________

2:00 _______________________

3:00 _______________________

4:00 _______________________

5:00 _______________________

6:00 _______________________

7:00 _______________________

8:00 _______________________

9:00 _______________________

10:00 ______________________

11:00 ______________________

Midnight ____________________

top priorities for today

____

____

____

____

Today's victories

What should you forgive
your self for?

____

____

____

____

____

____

The Stella Society Training

Exercise	Set 1	Set 2	Set 3	Set 4	Set 5	notes

Time started: ______________ Time ended: ______________

Location: ____

Feelings before training:        

Feelings after training

NUTRITION

Meal 1

time eaten: _________

Meal 2

time eaten: _________

Meal 3

time eaten: _________

Meal 4

time eaten: _________

Meal 5

time eaten: _________

Hydration

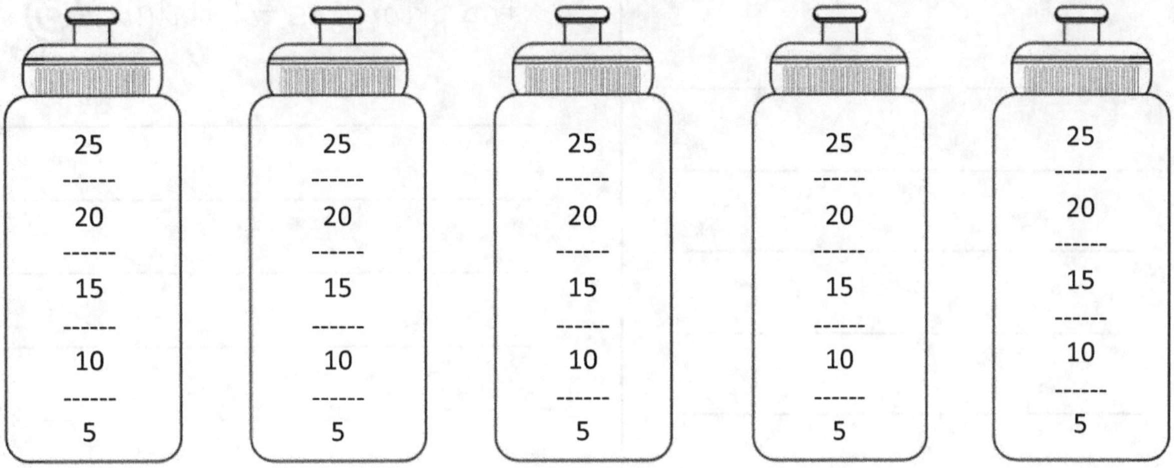

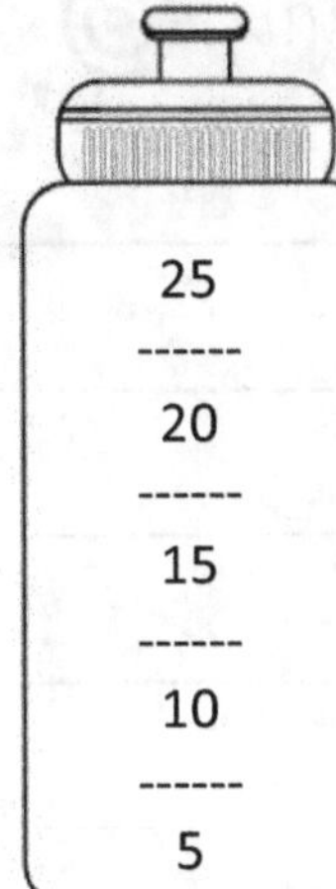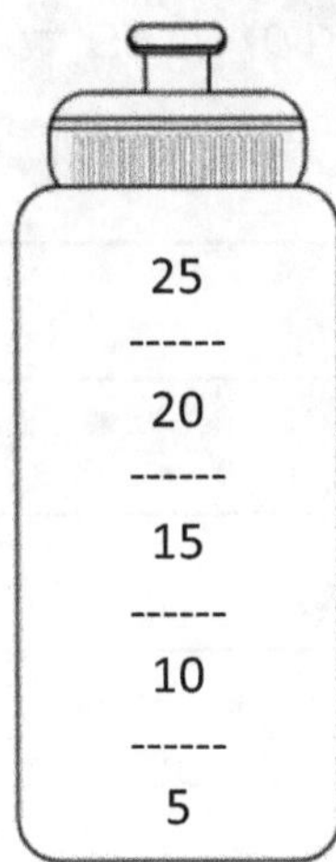

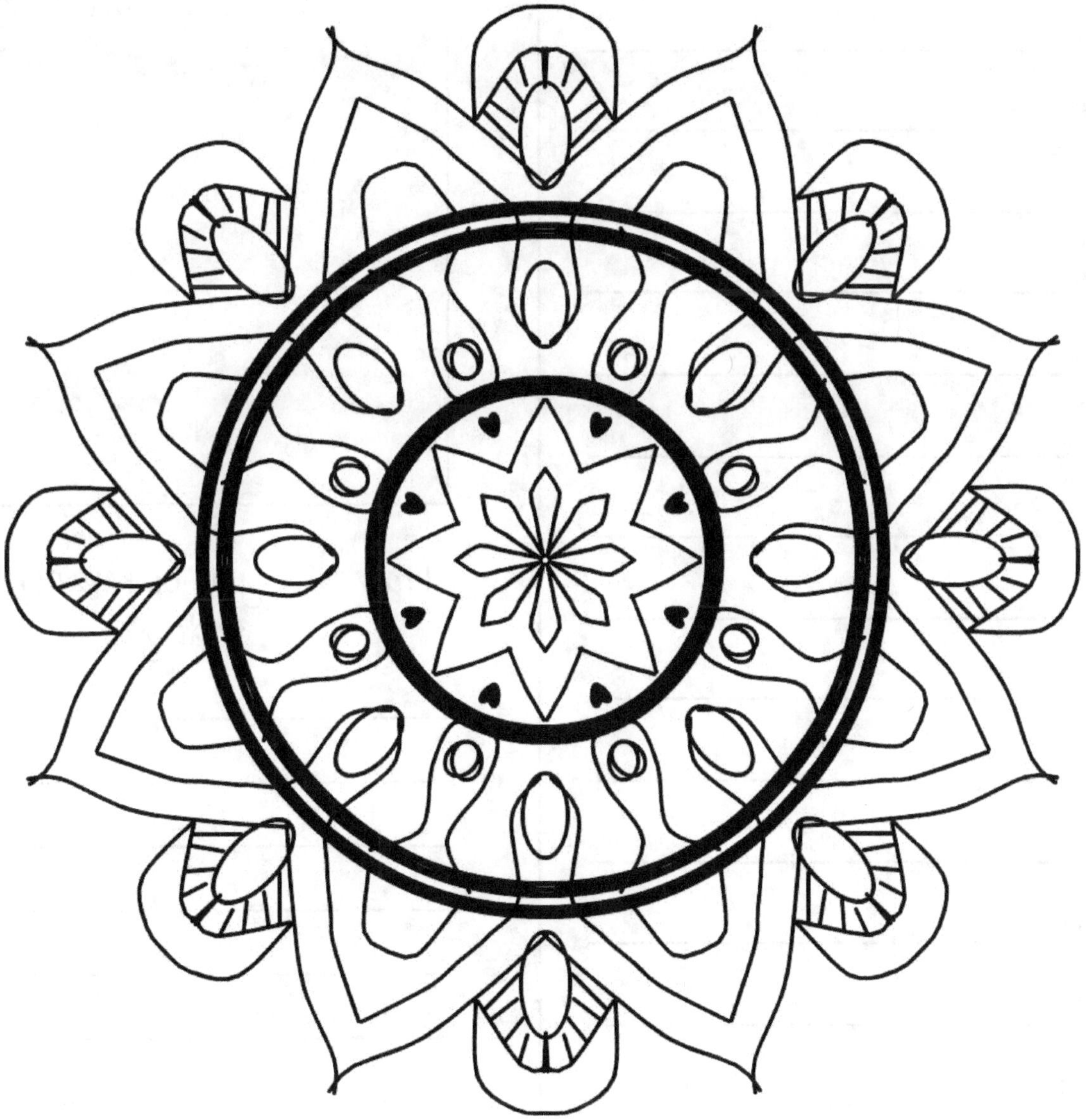

Day Fifteen _______

5:00 _______________________

6:00 _______________________

7:00 _______________________

8:00 _______________________

9:00 _______________________

10:00 ______________________

11:00 ______________________

Noon _______________________

1:00 _______________________

2:00 _______________________

3:00 _______________________

4:00 _______________________

5:00 _______________________

6:00 _______________________

7:00 _______________________

8:00 _______________________

9:00 _______________________

10:00 ______________________

11:00 ______________________

Midnight ___________________

top priorities for today

____

____

____

____

Today's victories

How will you be remarkable today?

____

____

____

____

____

____

The Training

Exercise	Set 1	Set 2	Set 3	Set 4	Set 5	notes

Time started: _____________ Time ended: _____________

Location: ____

Feelings before training: 🙂 😑 🙁 😜 😠 😕 😊 😎

Feelings after training 🙂 😑 🙁 😜 😠 😕 😊 😎

NUTRITION

Meal 1

time eaten: _________

Meal 2

time eaten: _________

Meal 3

time eaten: _________

Meal 4

time eaten: _________

Meal 5

time eaten: _________

Hydration

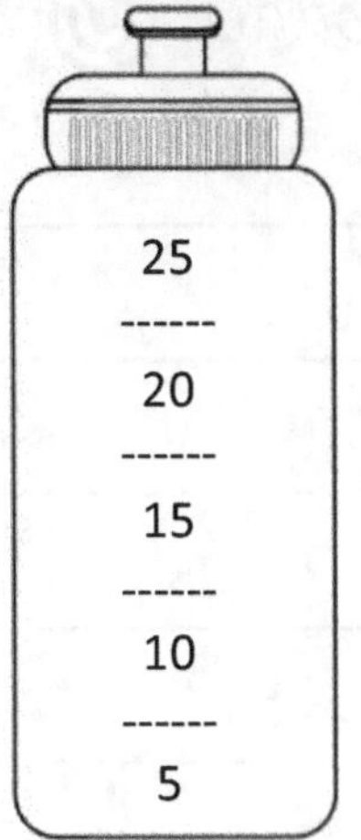

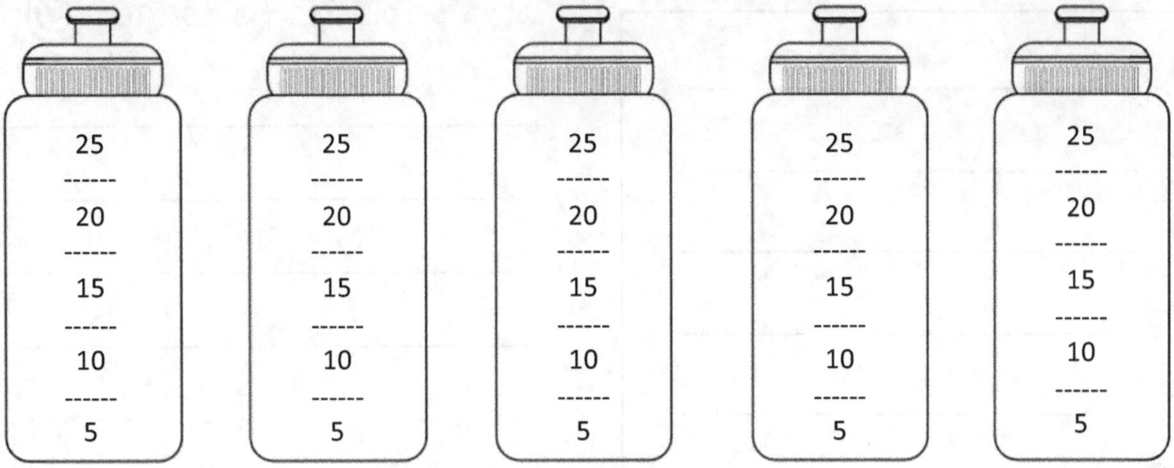

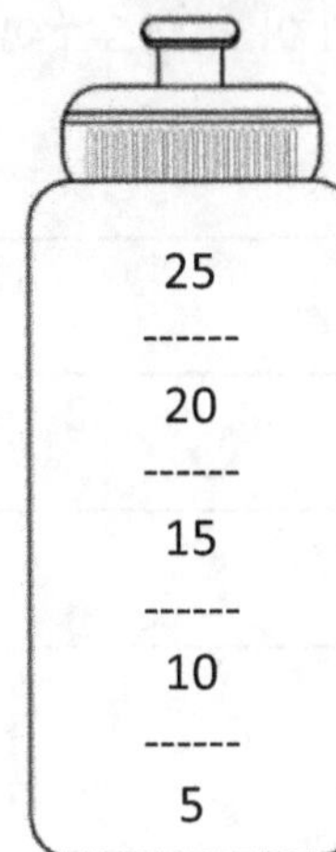

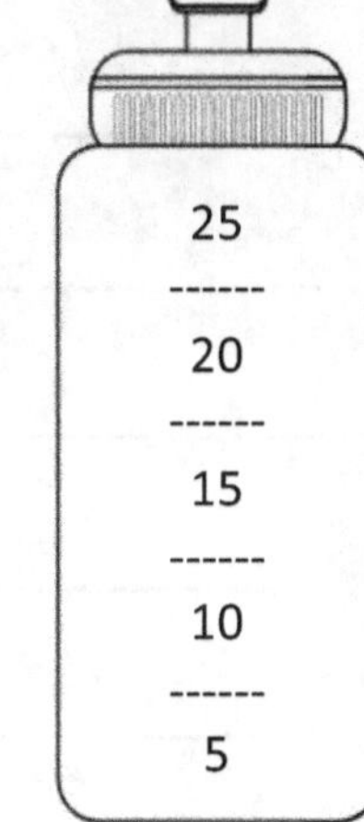

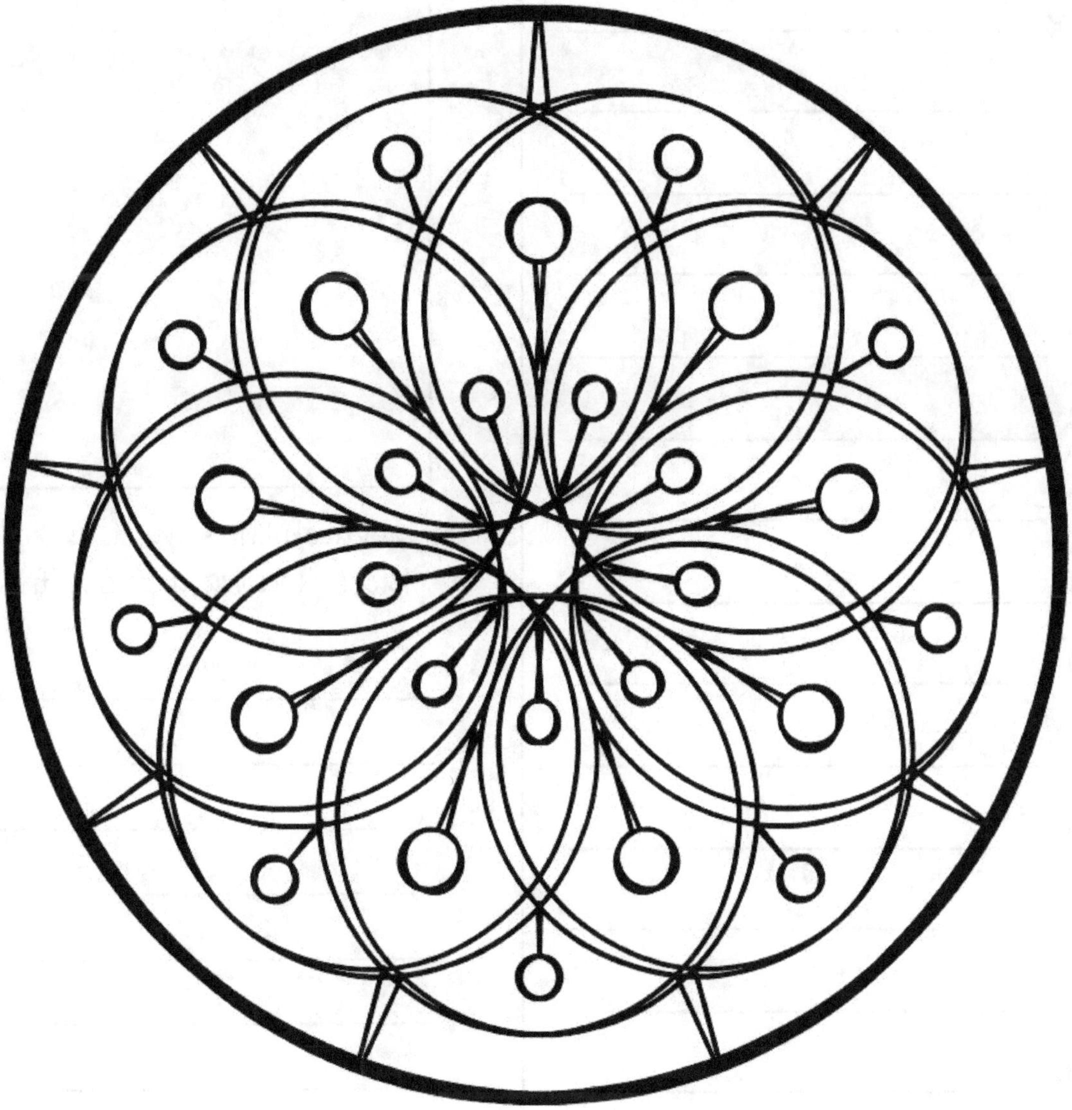

Day Sixteen __________

top priorities for today

5:00	__________
6:00	__________
7:00	__________
8:00	__________
9:00	__________
10:00	__________
11:00	__________
Noon	__________
1:00	__________
2:00	__________
3:00	__________
4:00	__________
5:00	__________
6:00	__________
7:00	__________
8:00	__________
9:00	__________
10:00	__________
11:00	__________
Midnight	__________

Today's victories

Watch the sunset and list 5 places you want to see it happen?

The Stella Society Training

Exercise	Set 1	Set 2	Set 3	Set 4	Set 5	notes

Time started: _____________ Time ended: _____________

Location: ____

Feelings before training:    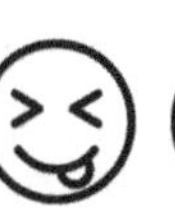   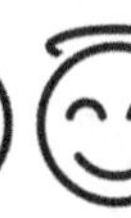  

Feelings after training

NUTRITION

Meal 1

time eaten: _________

Meal 2

time eaten: _________

Meal 3

time eaten: _________

Meal 4

time eaten: _________

Meal 5

time eaten: _________

Hydration

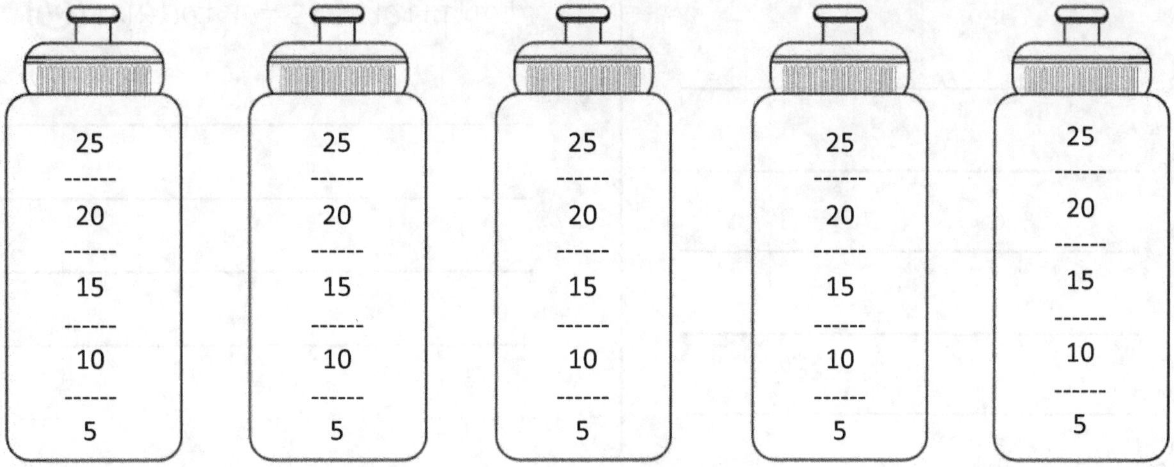

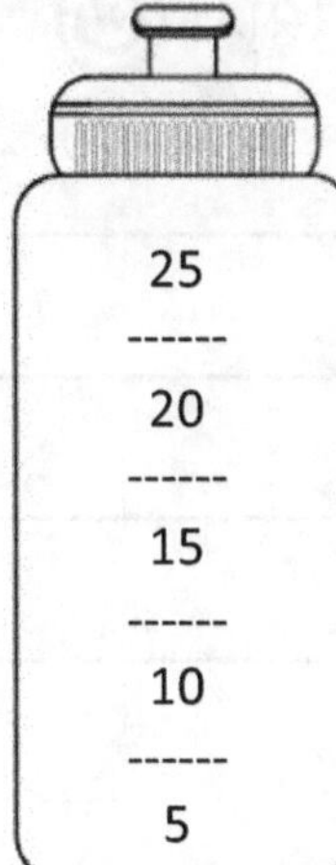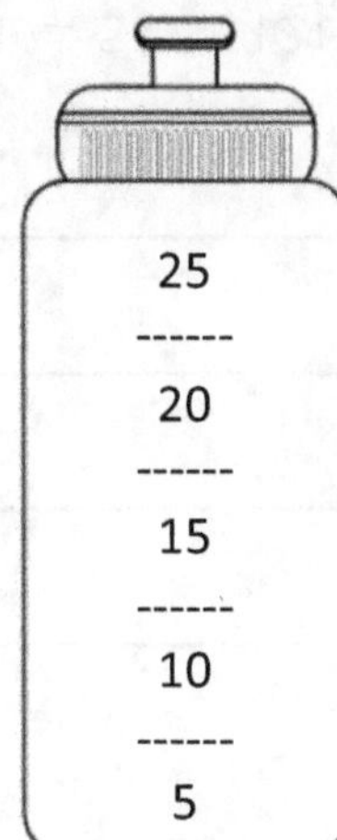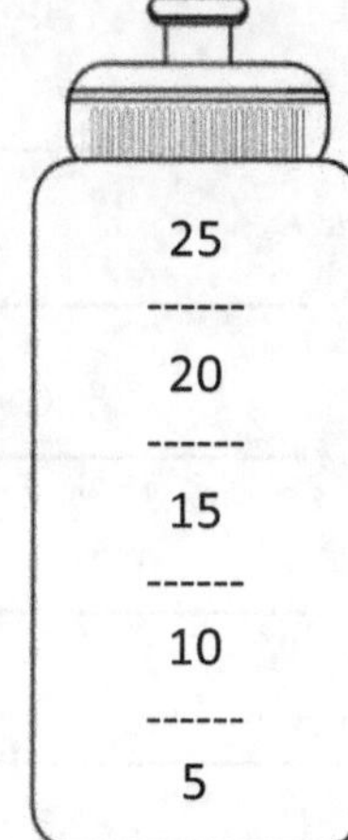

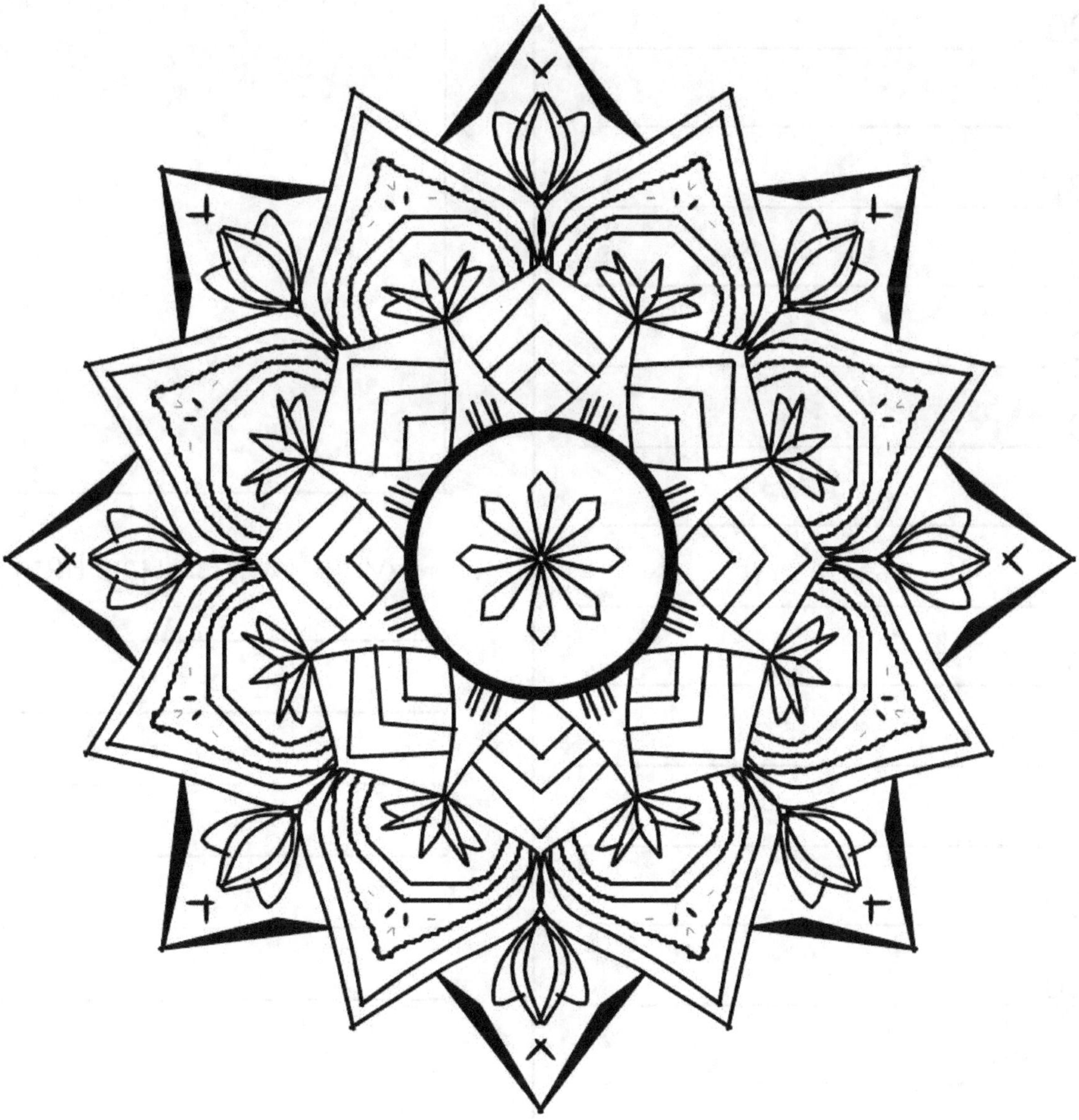

Day Seventeen ______

5:00 ______________________

6:00 ______________________

7:00 ______________________

8:00 ______________________

9:00 ______________________

10:00 _____________________

11:00 _____________________

Noon ______________________

1:00 ______________________

2:00 ______________________

3:00 ______________________

4:00 ______________________

5:00 ______________________

6:00 ______________________

7:00 ______________________

8:00 ______________________

9:00 ______________________

10:00 _____________________

11:00 _____________________

Midnight ___________________

top priorities for today

____

____

____

____

Today's victories

What makes you happy?

____

____

____

____

____

____

The Stella Society Training

Exercise	Set 1	Set 2	Set 3	Set 4	Set 5	notes

Time started: _______________ Time ended: _______________

Location: ____

Feelings before training: 

Feelings after training

NUTRITION

Meal 1

time eaten: _________

Meal 2

time eaten: _________

Meal 3

time eaten: _________

Meal 4

time eaten: _________

Meal 5

time eaten: _________

Hydration

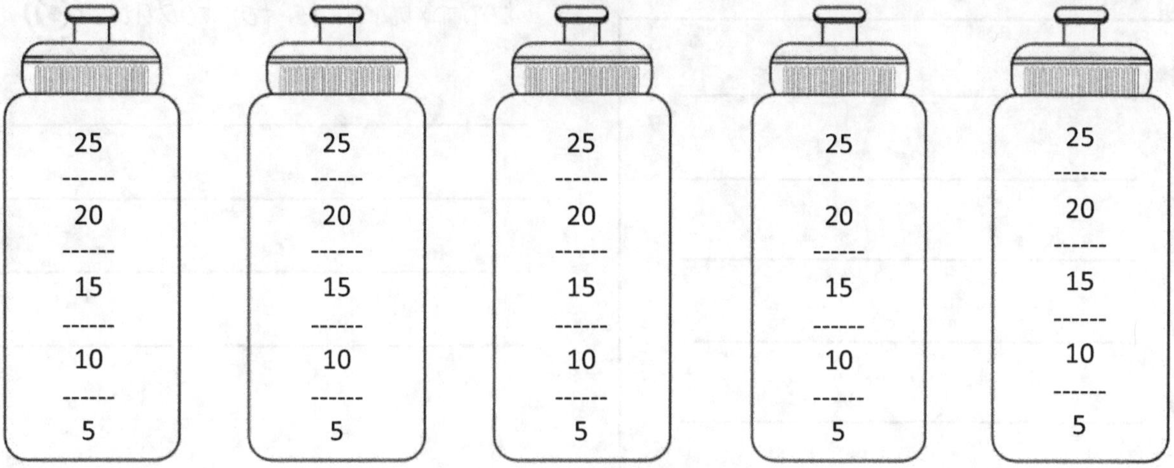

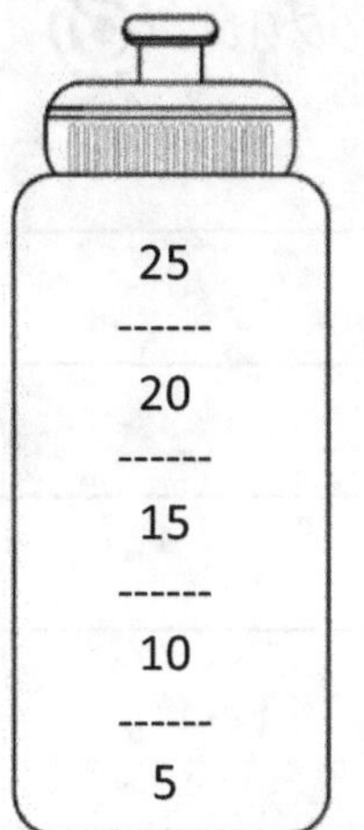 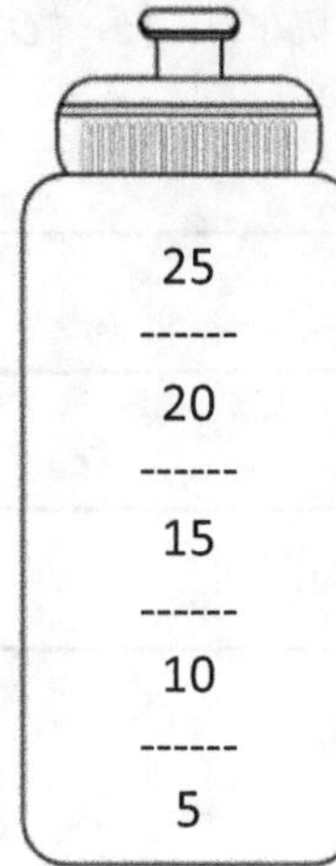 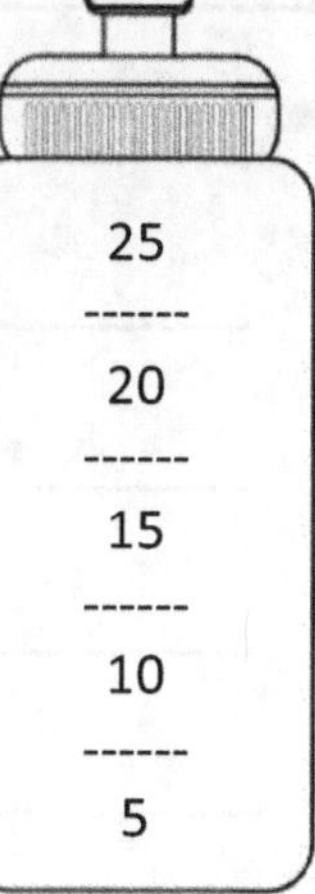

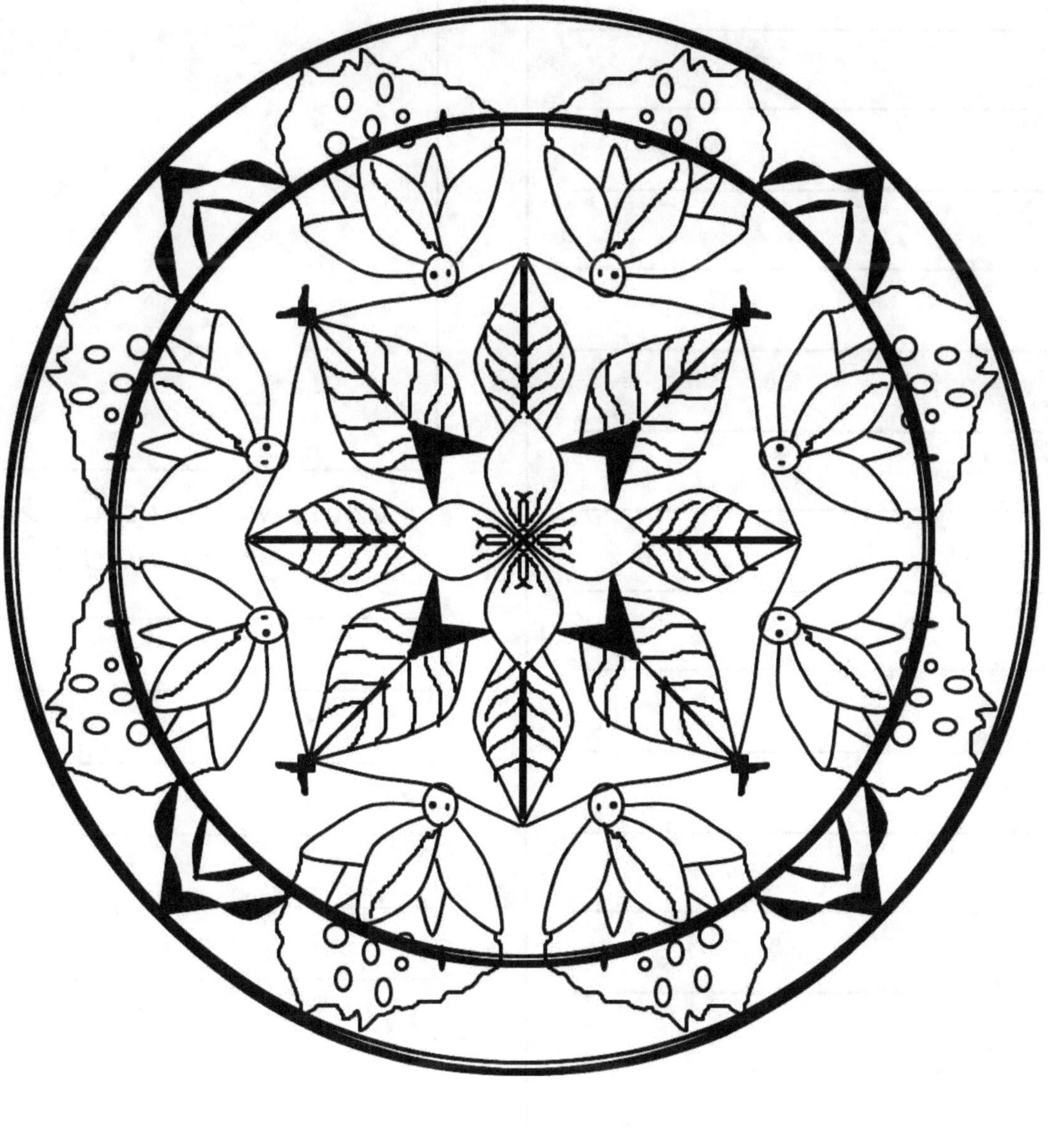

Day Eighteen ________

5:00 ______________________

6:00 ______________________

7:00 ______________________

8:00 ______________________

9:00 ______________________

10:00 ______________________

11:00 ______________________

Noon ______________________

1:00 ______________________

2:00 ______________________

3:00 ______________________

4:00 ______________________

5:00 ______________________

6:00 ______________________

7:00 ______________________

8:00 ______________________

9:00 ______________________

10:00 ______________________

11:00 ______________________

Midnight __________________

Today's victories

Where will you shine your
light this week?

The Stella Society Training

Exercise	Set 1	Set 2	Set 3	Set 4	Set 5	notes

Time started: _____________ Time ended: _____________

Location: ____

Feelings before training:

Feelings after training

NUTRITION

Meal 1
time eaten: _________

Meal 2
time eaten: _________

Meal 3
time eaten: _________

Meal 4
time eaten: _________

Meal 5
time eaten: _________

Hydration

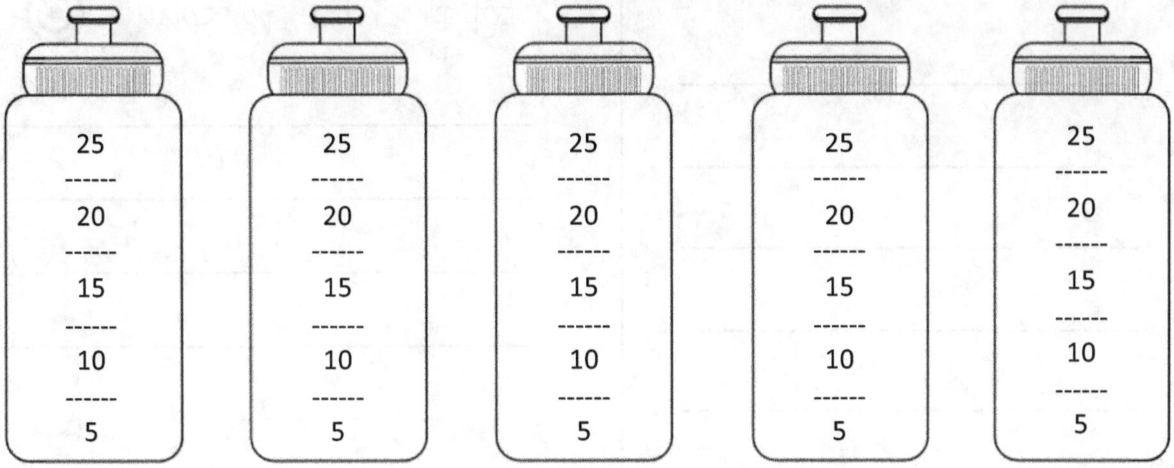

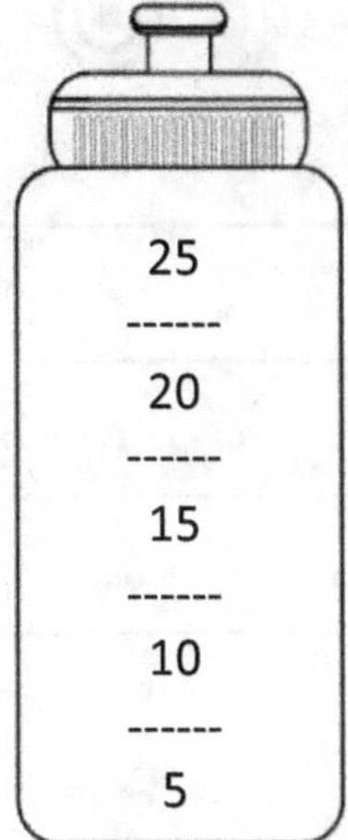 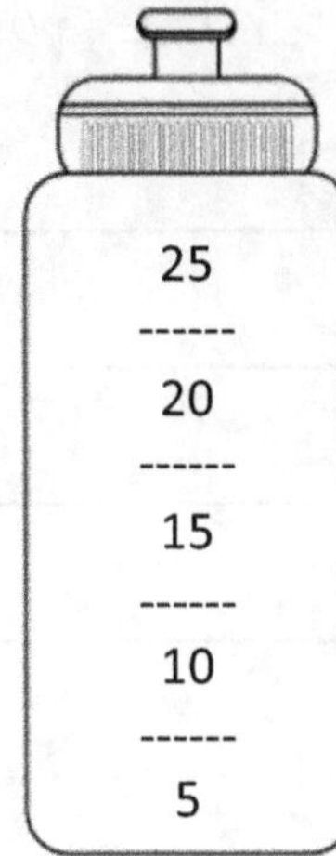

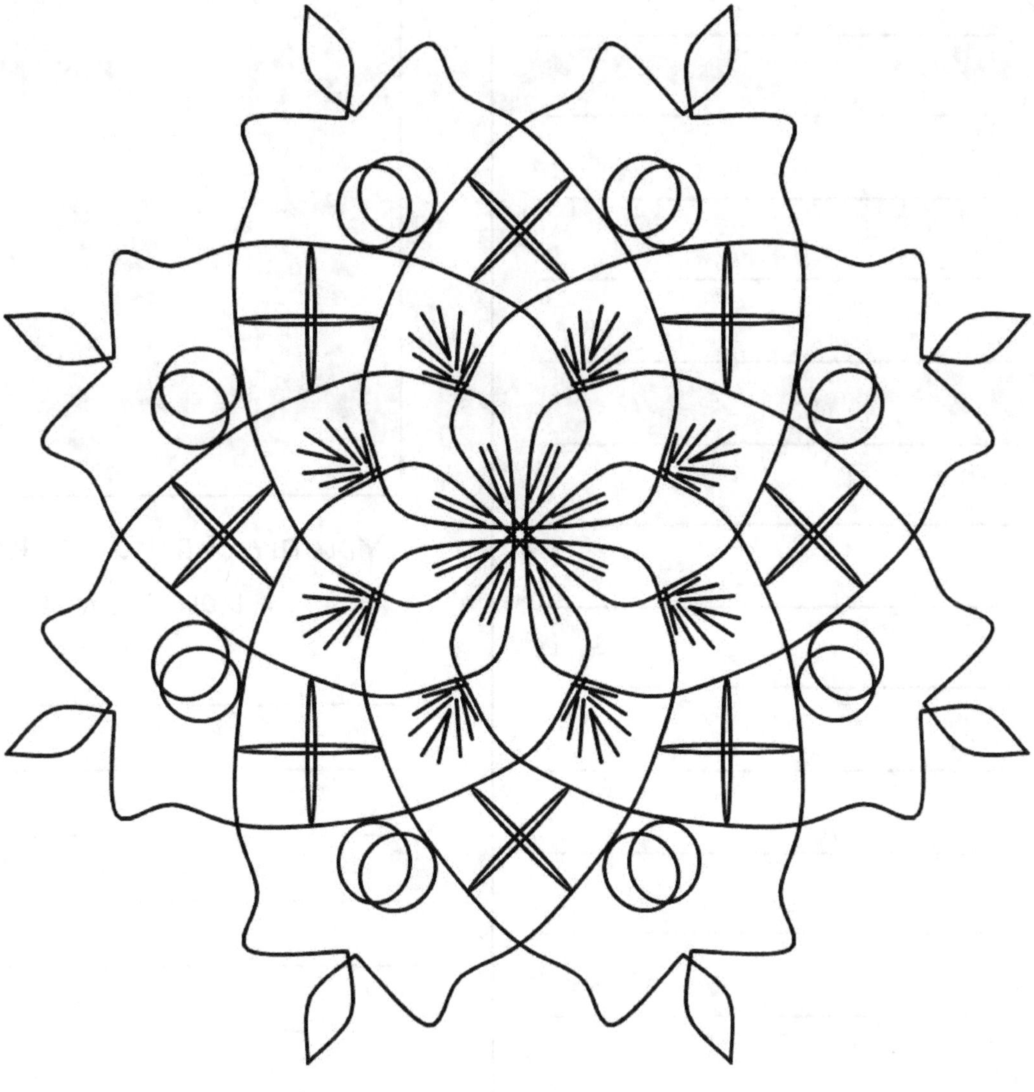

Day Nineteen _______

5:00 _______________

6:00 _______________

7:00 _______________

8:00 _______________

9:00 _______________

10:00 _______________

11:00 _______________

Noon _______________

1:00 _______________

2:00 _______________

3:00 _______________

4:00 _______________

5:00 _______________

6:00 _______________

7:00 _______________

8:00 _______________

9:00 _______________

10:00 _______________

11:00 _______________

Midnight _______________

____

____

____

____

You are charming, how will you show it?

____

____

____

____

____

____

The Training

Exercise	Set 1	Set 2	Set 3	Set 4	Set 5	notes

Time started: _____________ Time ended: ______________

Location: ____

Feelings before training:

Feelings after training

NUTRITION

Meal 1

time eaten: _________

Meal 2

time eaten: _________

Meal 3

time eaten: _________

Meal 4

time eaten: _________

Meal 5

time eaten: _________

Hydration

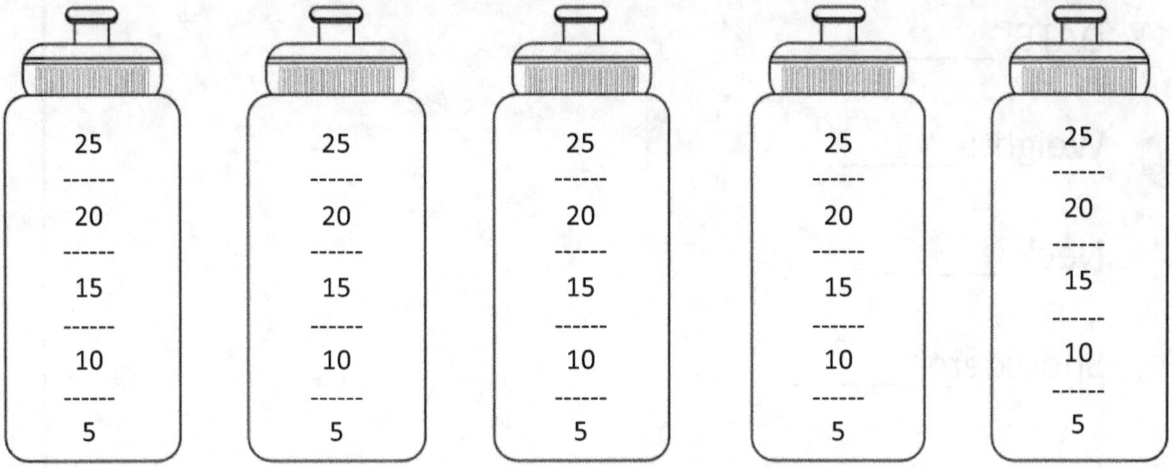

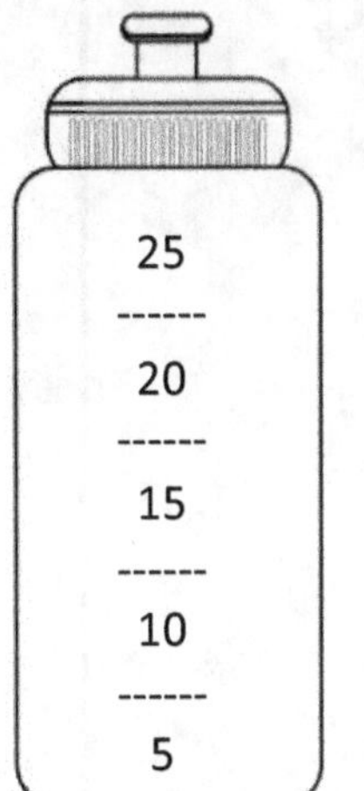 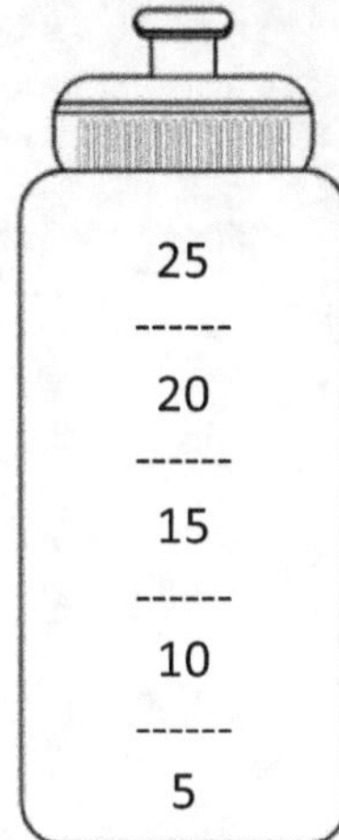

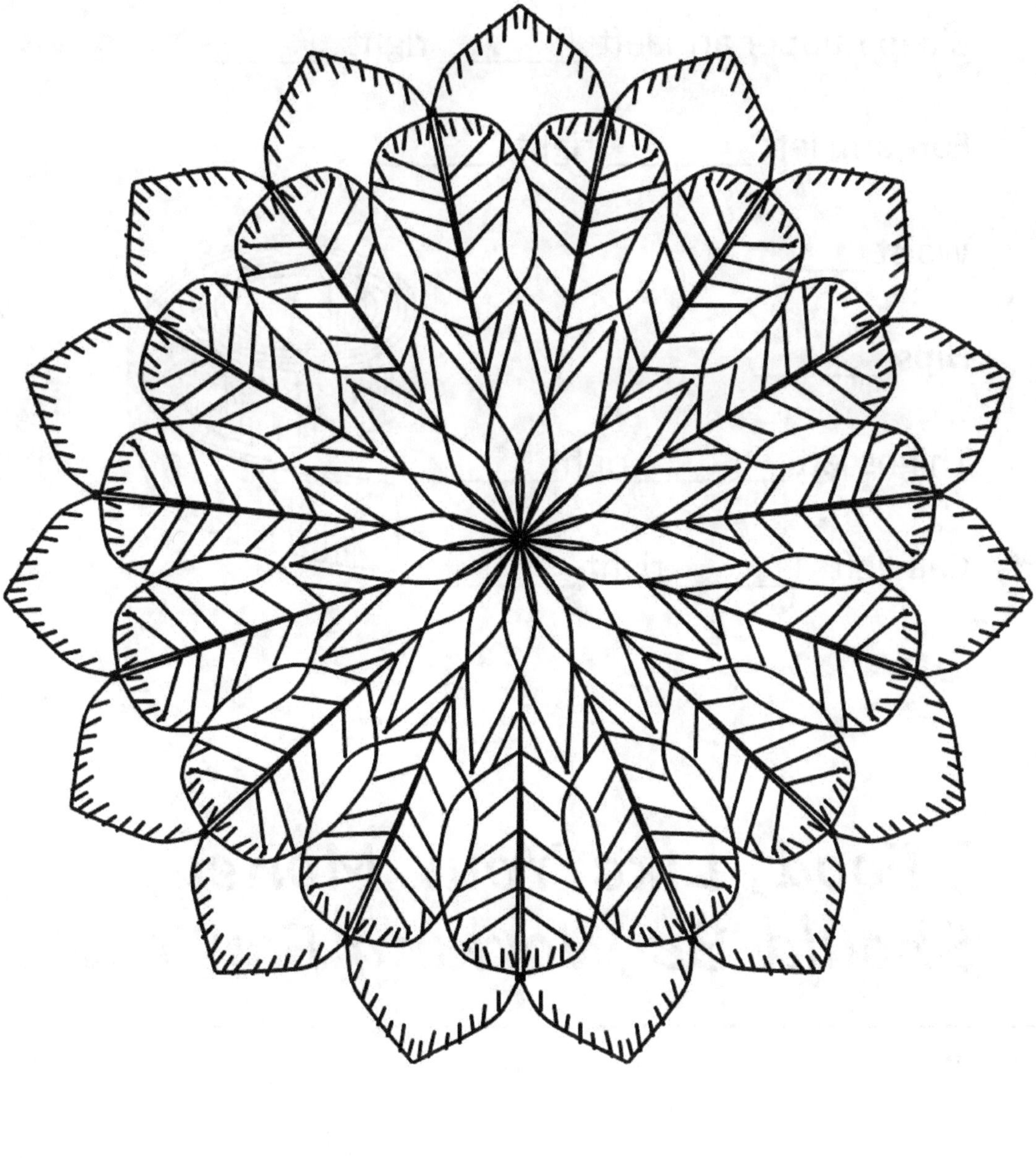

Measurements

DATE: _________

Weight: ______

Neck ______

Shoulders ______

Chest ______

Bicep / upper arm left ________ right ______

Forearm left _______ right _______

Waist ______

Hips ______

Thighs left _______ right ______

Calf left _______ right _______

Food, Like Your Money,
Should Be Working For You

Day Twenty _______

5:00 _______________________

6:00 _______________________

7:00 _______________________

8:00 _______________________

9:00 _______________________

10:00 ______________________

11:00 ______________________

Noon _______________________

1:00 _______________________

2:00 _______________________

3:00 _______________________

4:00 _______________________

5:00 _______________________

6:00 _______________________

7:00 _______________________

8:00 _______________________

9:00 _______________________

10:00 ______________________

11:00 ______________________

Midnight ___________________

top priorities for today 🎯

____

____

____

____

Today's victories 🏆

What is your level of understanding difficult situations?

____

____

____

____

____

The Stella Society Workout

Exercise	Set 1	Set 2	Set 3	Set 4	Set 5	notes

Time started: ______________   Time ended: ______________

Location: ____

Feelings before training:

Feelings after training

NUTRITION

Meal 1

time eaten: _________

Meal 2

time eaten: _________

Meal 3

time eaten: _________

Meal 4

time eaten: _________

Meal 5

time eaten: _________

Hydration

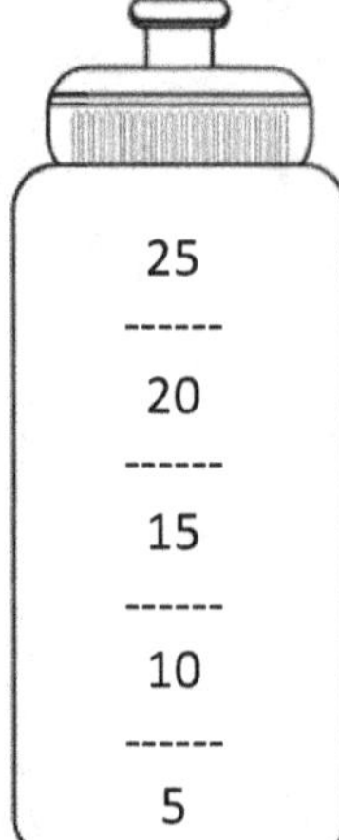

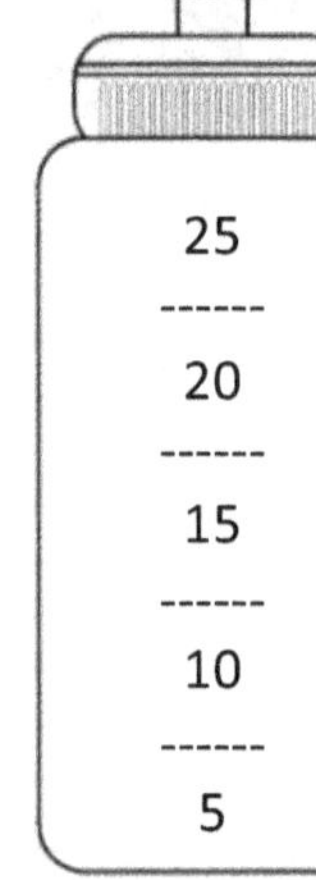

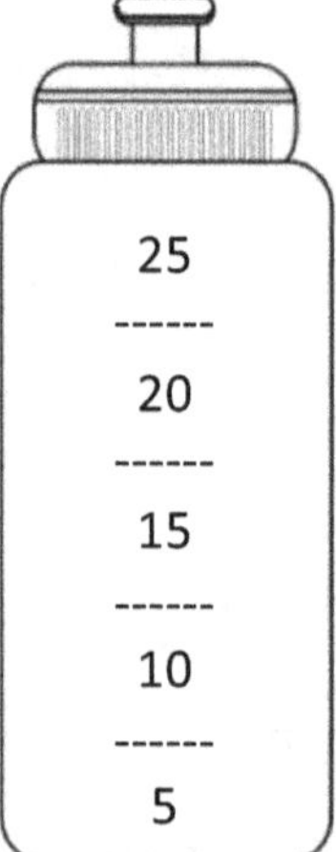

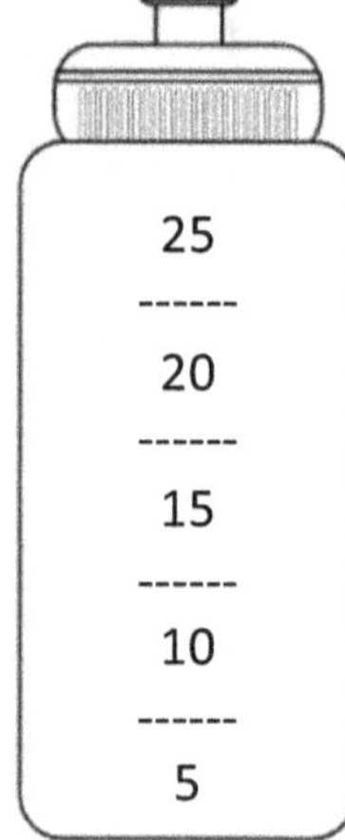

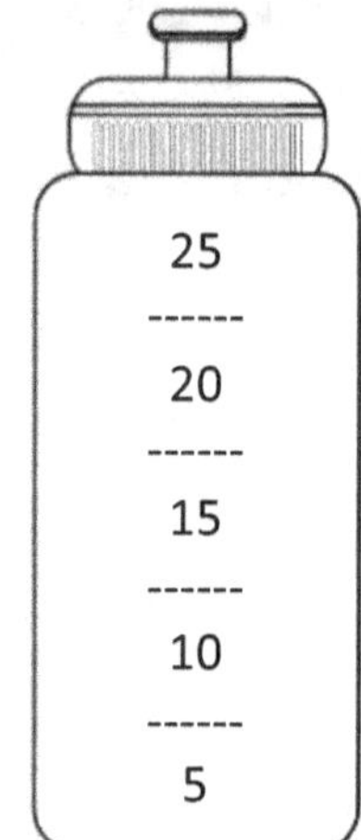

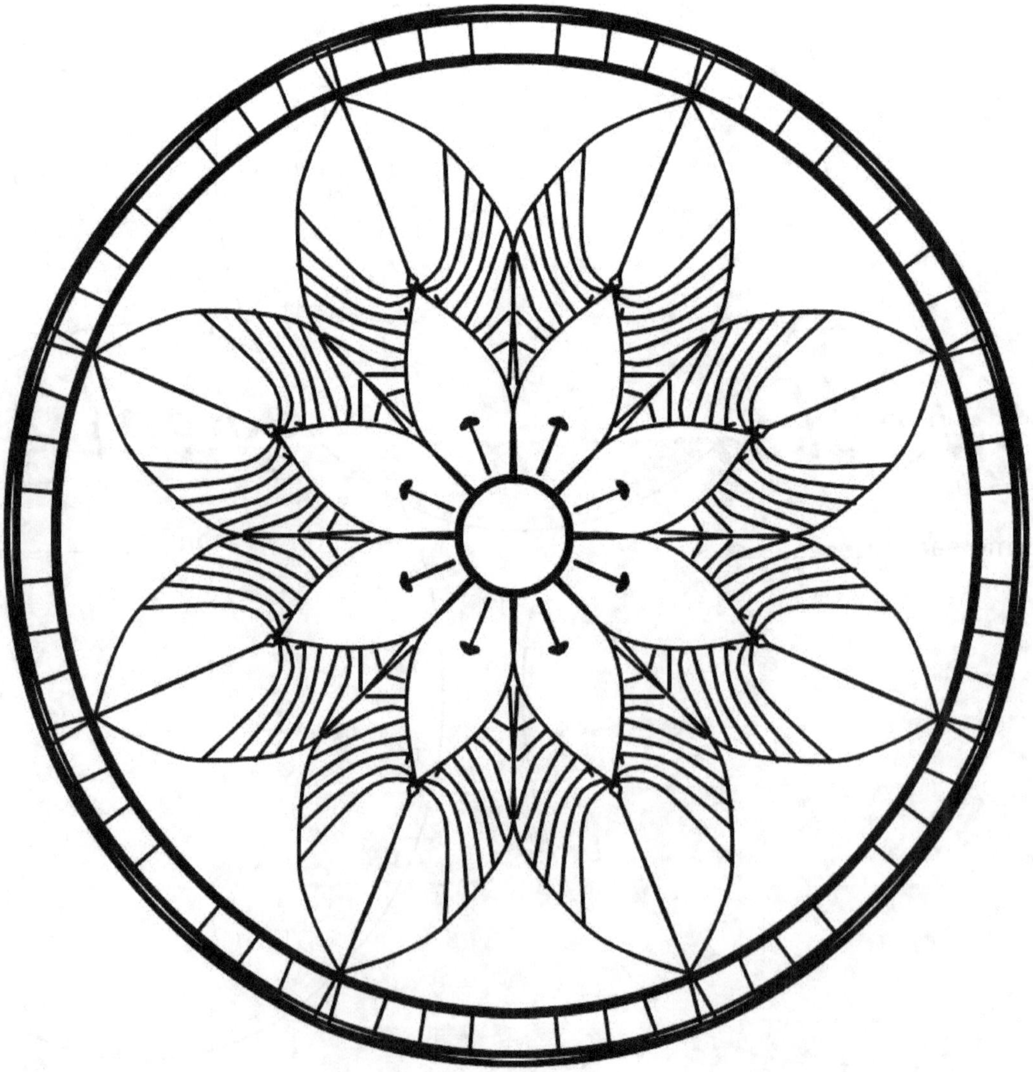

Day Twenty-one _______

Time	
5:00	_________________
6:00	_________________
7:00	_________________
8:00	_________________
9:00	_________________
10:00	_________________
11:00	_________________
Noon	_________________
1:00	_________________
2:00	_________________
3:00	_________________
4:00	_________________
5:00	_________________
6:00	_________________
7:00	_________________
8:00	_________________
9:00	_________________
10:00	_________________
11:00	_________________
Midnight	_________________

top priorities for today

____
____
____
____
____

Today's victories

How much can you endure?

____
____
____
____
____
____
____

The Stella Society Workout

Exercise	Set 1	Set 2	Set 3	Set 4	Set 5	notes

Time started: _____________ Time ended: _____________

Location: ____

Feelings before training:

Feelings after training

NUTRITION

Meal 1
time eaten: _________

Meal 2
time eaten: _________

Meal 3
time eaten: _________

Meal 4
time eaten: _________

Meal 5
time eaten: _________

Hydration

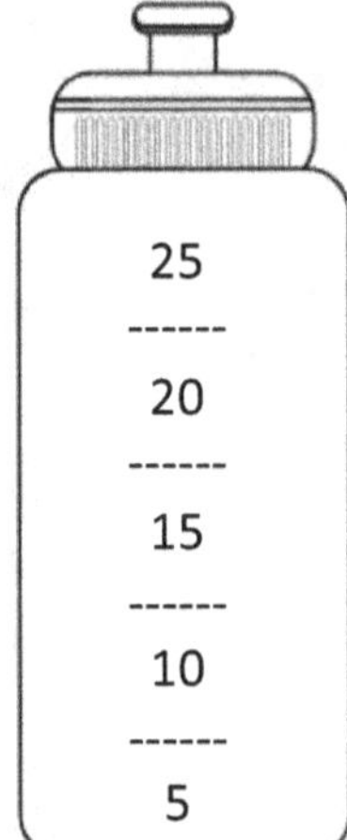 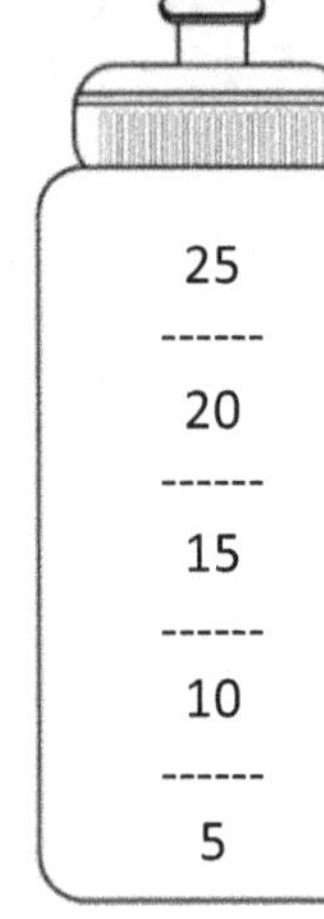 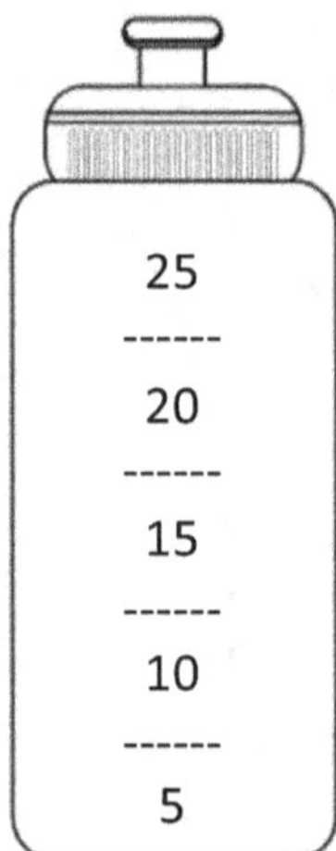 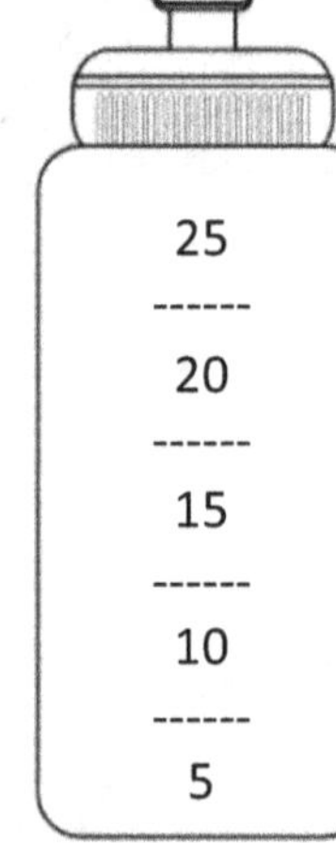 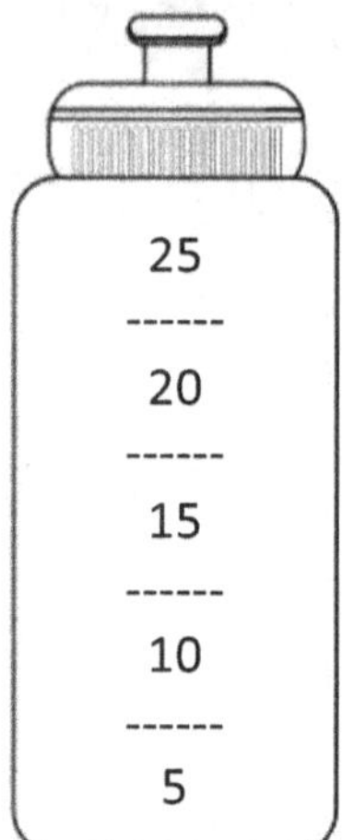

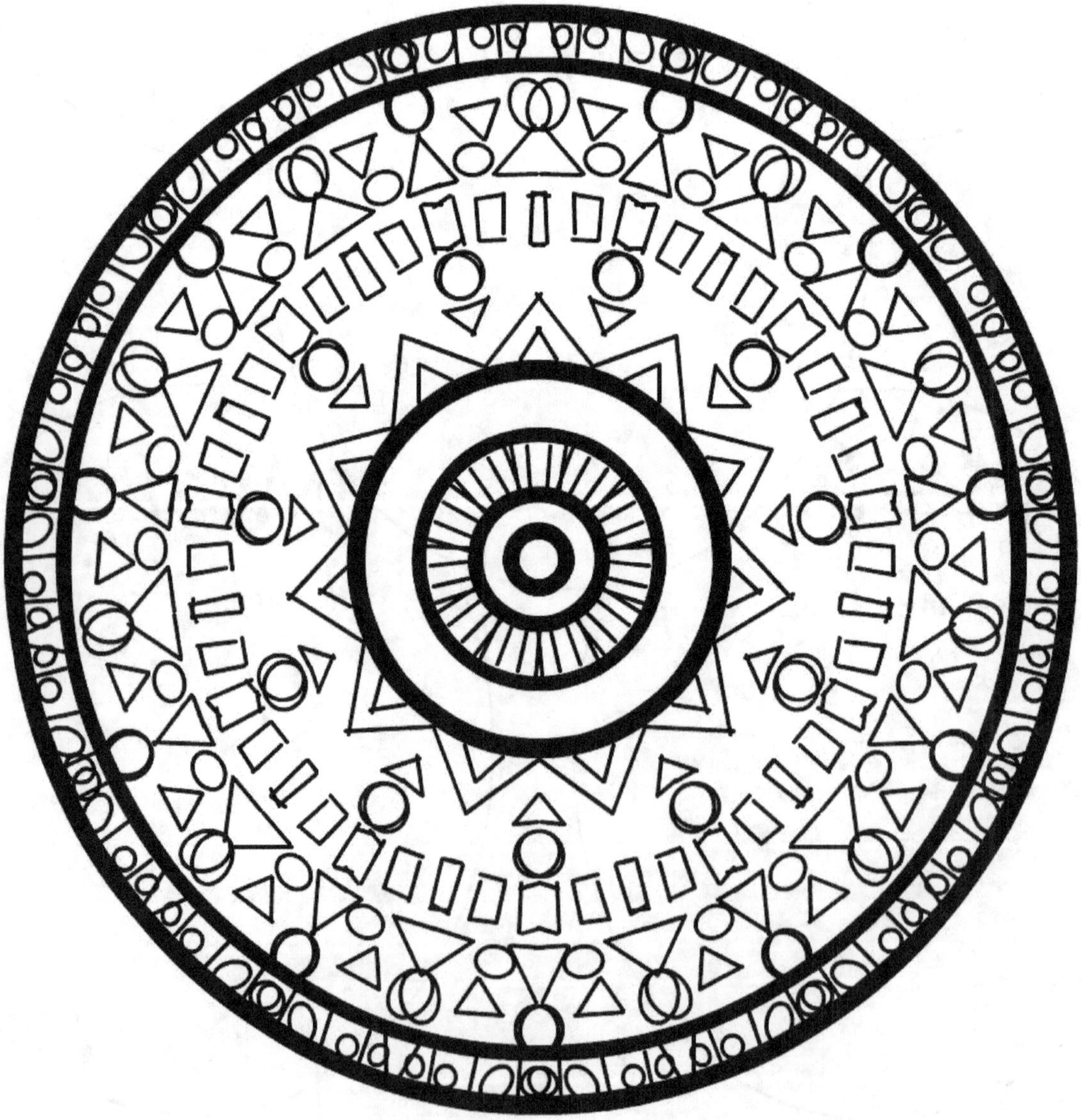

Day Twenty-two __________

5:00 __________________

6:00 __________________

7:00 __________________

8:00 __________________

9:00 __________________

10:00 __________________

11:00 __________________

Noon __________________

1:00 __________________

2:00 __________________

3:00 __________________

4:00 __________________

5:00 __________________

6:00 __________________

7:00 __________________

8:00 __________________

9:00 __________________

10:00 __________________

11:00 __________________

Midnight __________________

top priorities for today

____

____

____

____

____

Today's victories

List 5 ways to be thoughtful.

____

____

____

____

____

____

____

The *Stella Society* Workout

Exercise	Set 1	Set 2	Set 3	Set 4	Set 5	notes

Time started: _____________   Time ended: _____________

Location: ____

Feelings before training:

Feelings after training

NUTRITION

Meal 1

time eaten: _________

Meal 2

time eaten: _________

Meal 3

time eaten: _________

Meal 4

time eaten: _________

Meal 5

time eaten: _________

Hydration

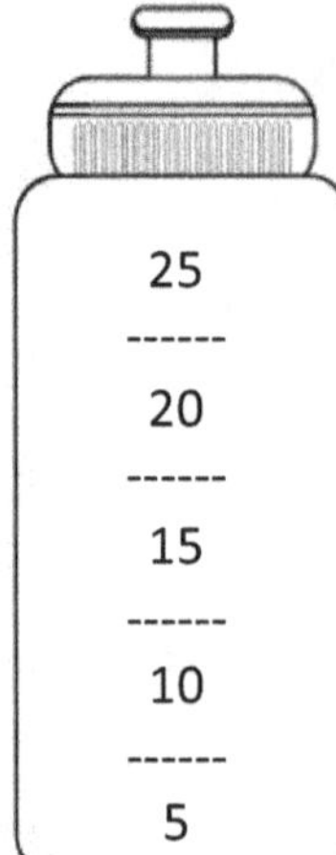
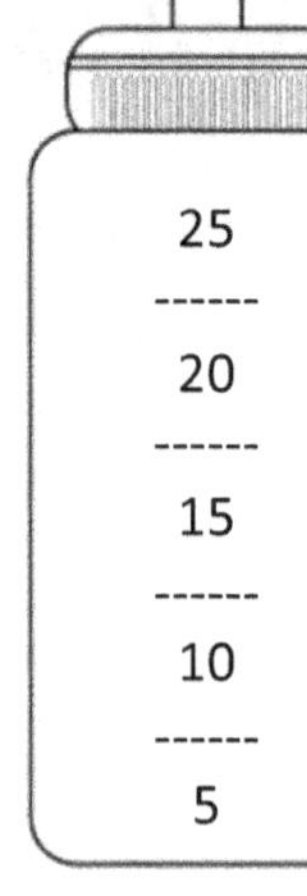
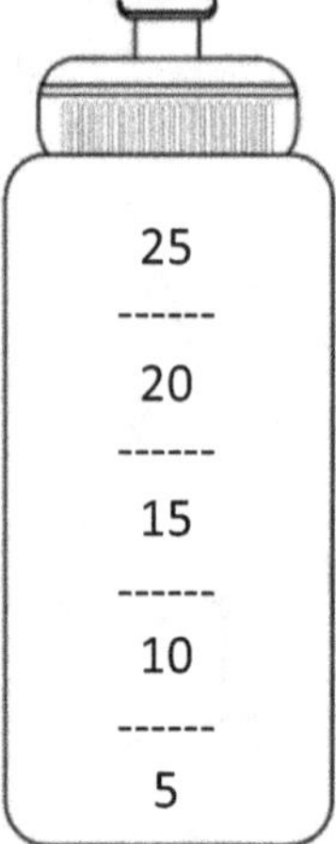
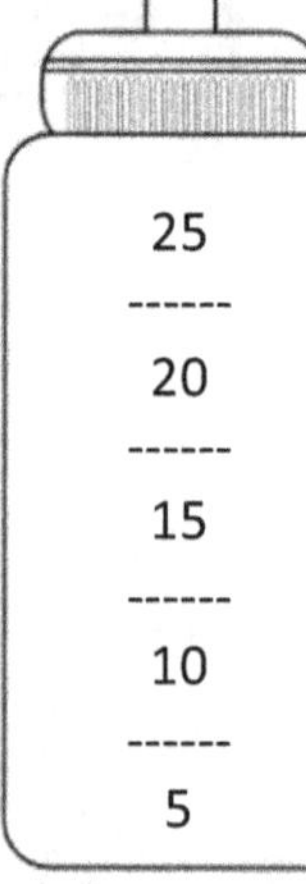
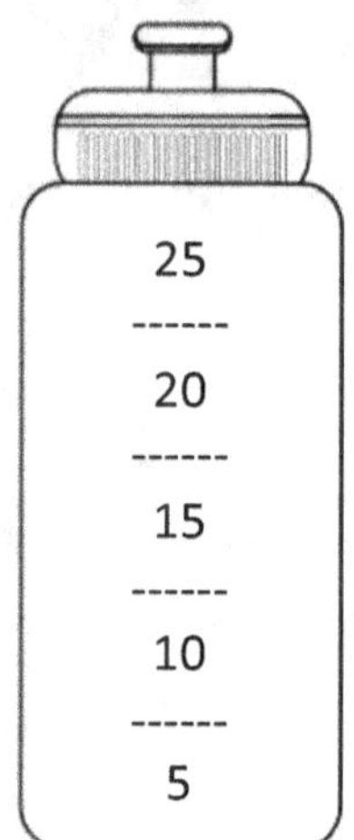

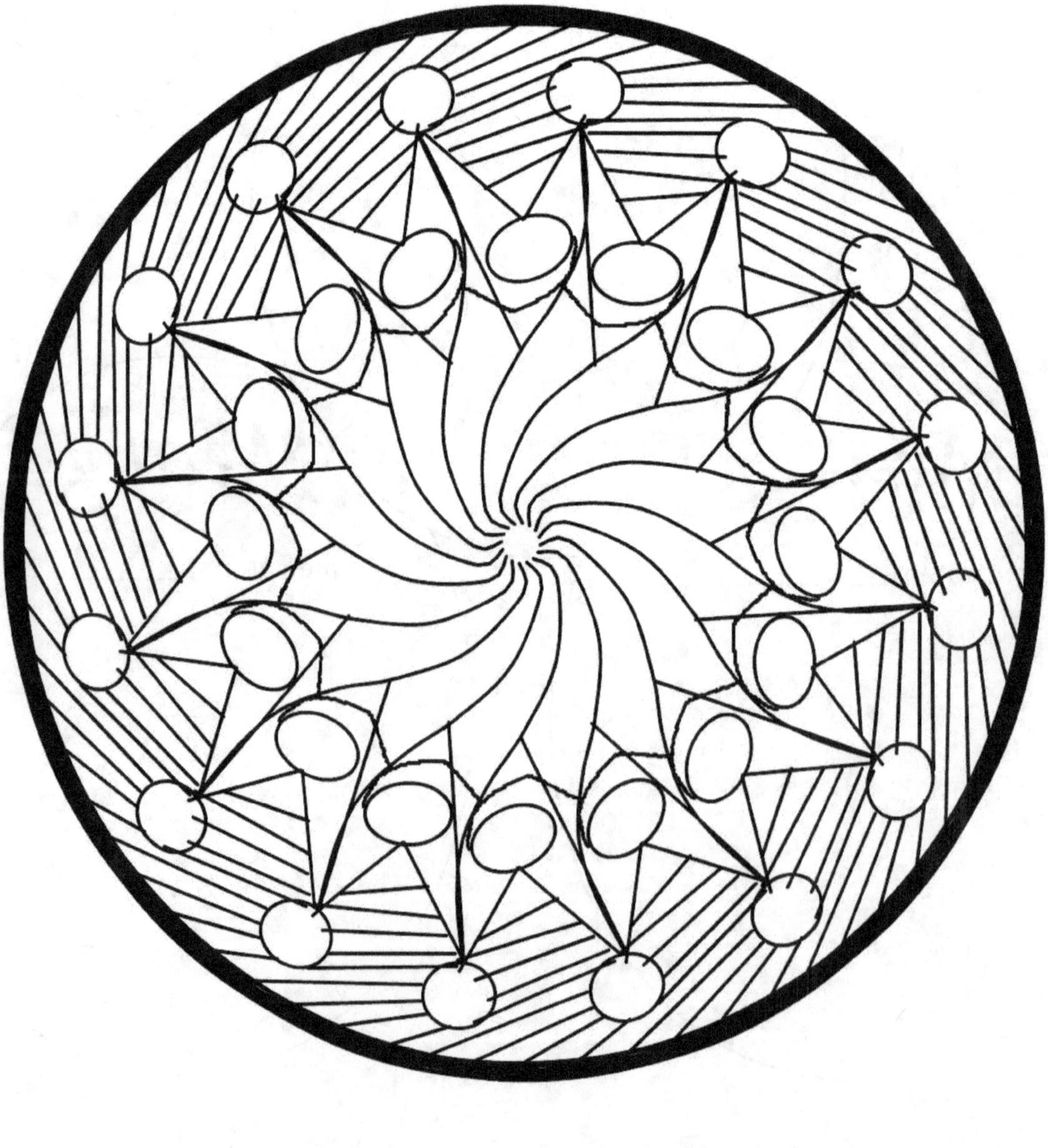

Day Twenty-three _______

5:00 ___________________

6:00 ___________________

7:00 ___________________

8:00 ___________________

9:00 ___________________

10:00 ___________________

11:00 ___________________

Noon ___________________

1:00 ___________________

2:00 ___________________

3:00 ___________________

4:00 ___________________

5:00 ___________________

6:00 ___________________

7:00 ___________________

8:00 ___________________

9:00 ___________________

10:00 ___________________

11:00 ___________________

Midnight ___________________

Today's victories

Why should you be unapologetic?

The Stella Society Workout

Exercise	Set 1	Set 2	Set 3	Set 4	Set 5	notes

Time started: _____________ Time ended: _____________

Location: ____

Feelings before training: 😊 😐 ☹ 😜 😠 😟 😇 😎

Feelings after training 😊 😐 ☹ 😜 😠 😟 😇 😎

NUTRITION

Meal 1

time eaten: _________

Meal 2

time eaten: _________

Meal 3

time eaten: _________

Meal 4

time eaten: _________

Meal 5

time eaten: _________

Hydration

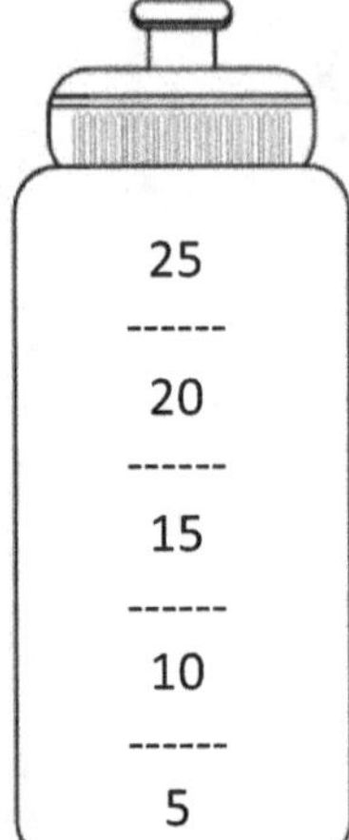

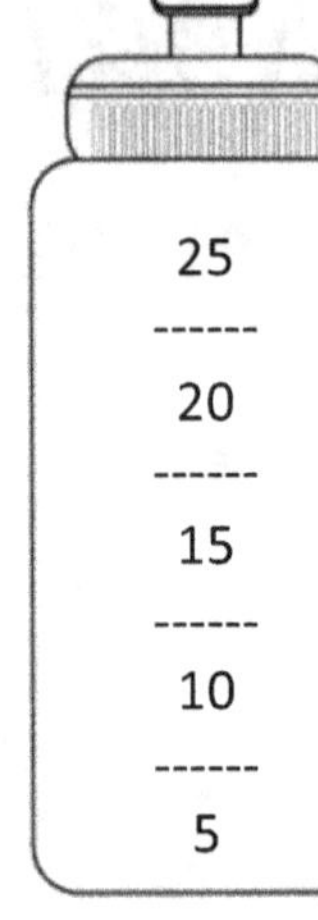

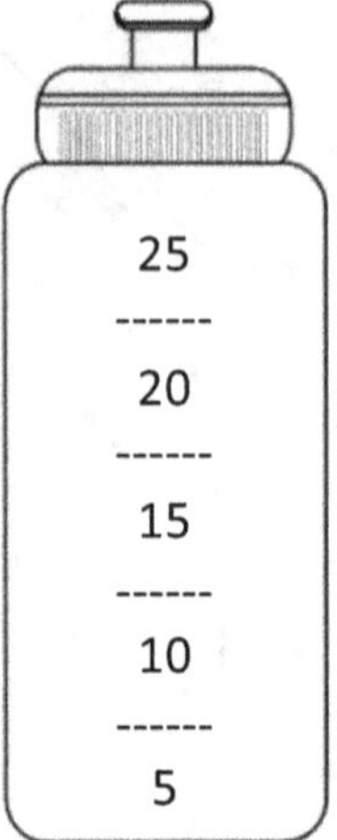

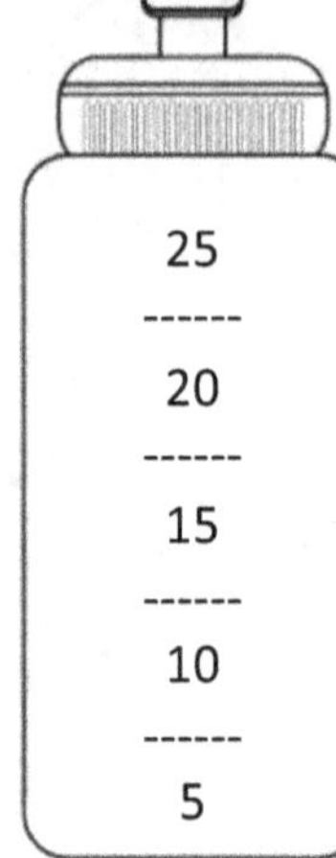

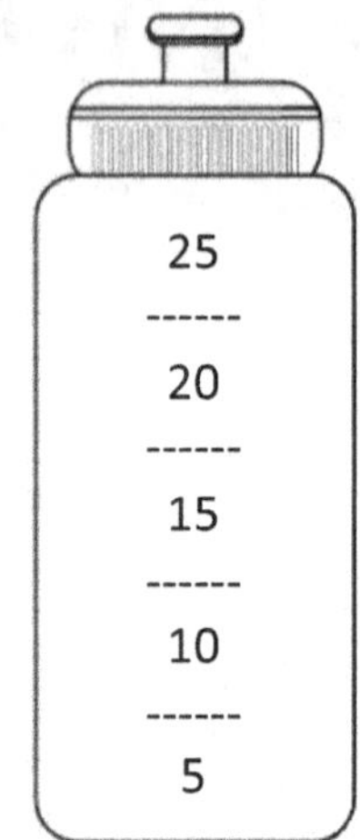

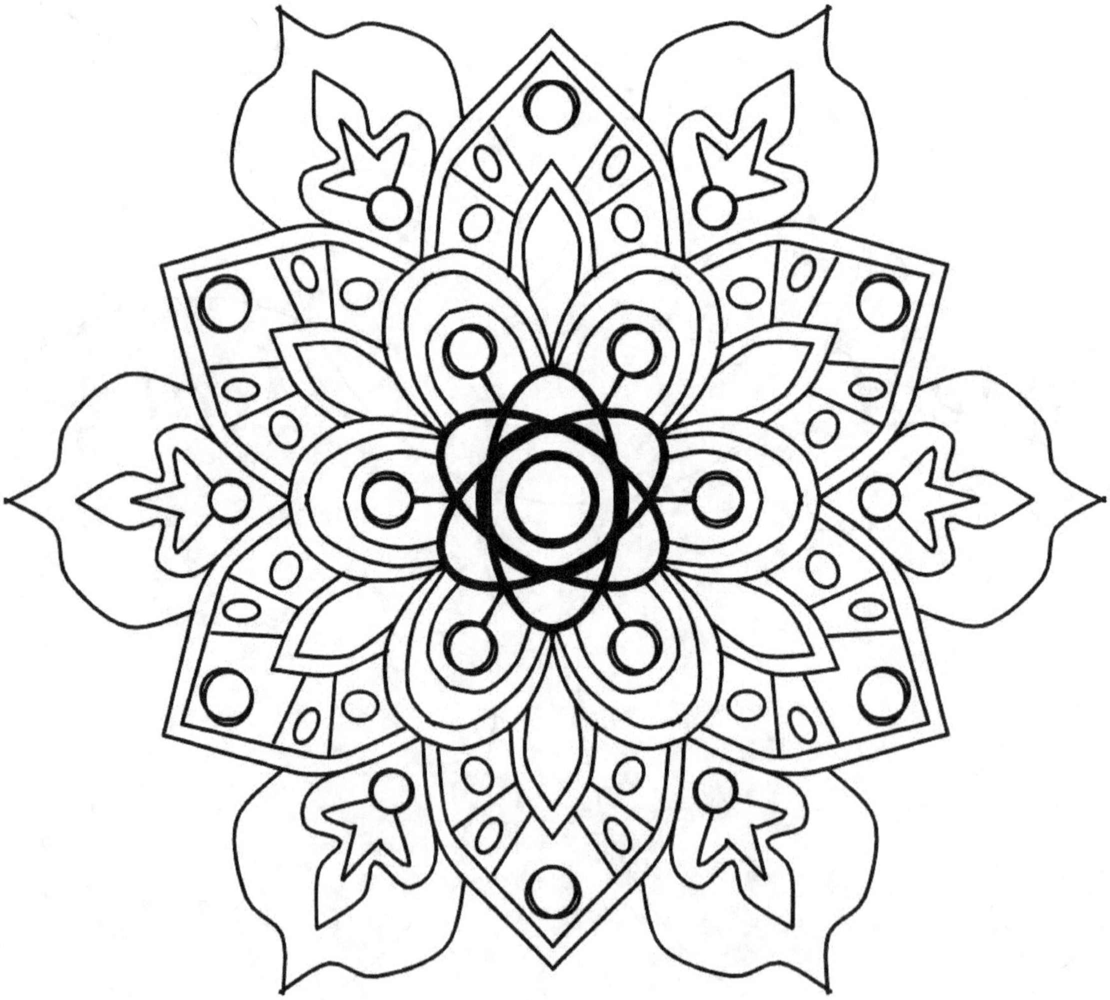

Day Twenty-four _______

5:00 _______________________

6:00 _______________________

7:00 _______________________

8:00 _______________________

9:00 _______________________

10:00 ______________________

11:00 ______________________

Noon _______________________

1:00 _______________________

2:00 _______________________

3:00 _______________________

4:00 _______________________

5:00 _______________________

6:00 _______________________

7:00 _______________________

8:00 _______________________

9:00 _______________________

10:00 ______________________

11:00 ______________________

Midnight ___________________

Today's victories

What can you set on fire
with your fierceness?

The Stella Society Workout

Exercise	Set 1	Set 2	Set 3	Set 4	Set 5	notes

Time started: _____________ Time ended: _____________

Location: ____

Feelings before training:

Feelings after training

NUTRITION

Meal 1

time eaten: _________

Meal 2

time eaten: _________

Meal 3

time eaten: _________

Meal 4

time eaten: _________

Meal 5

time eaten: _________

Hydration

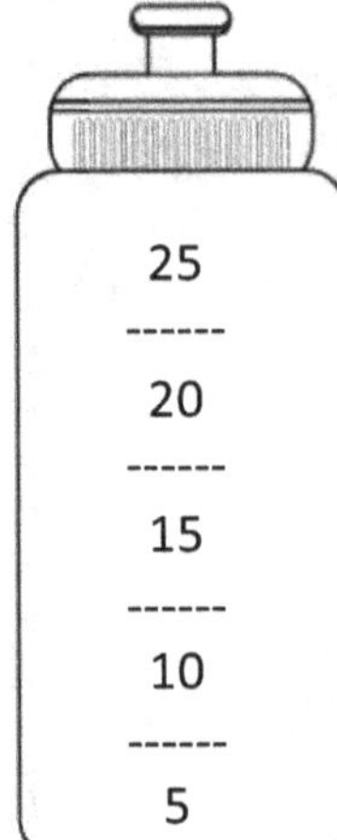 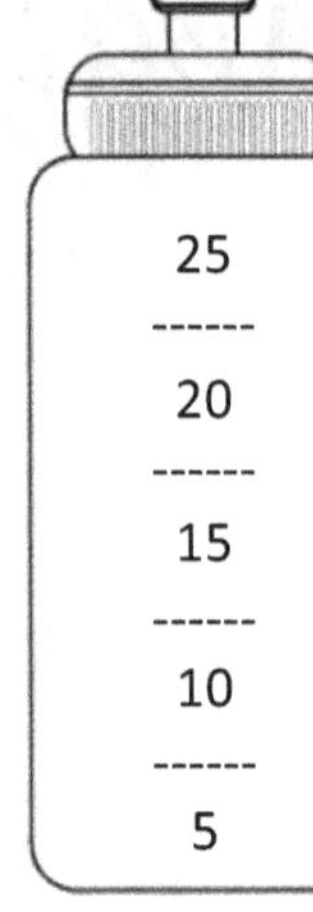 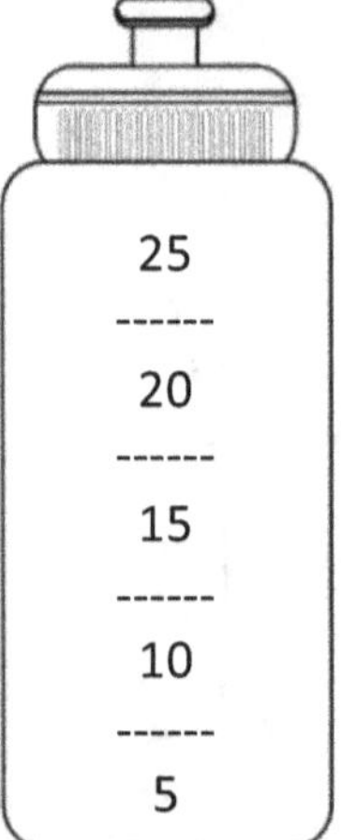 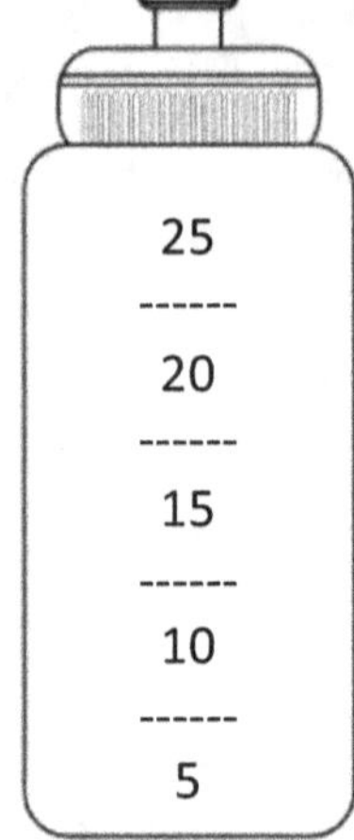 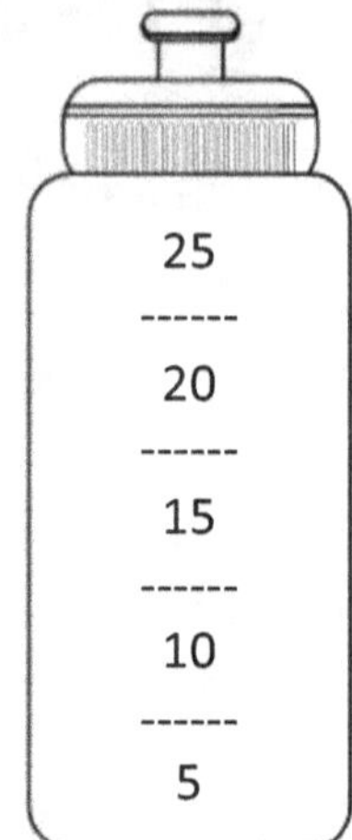

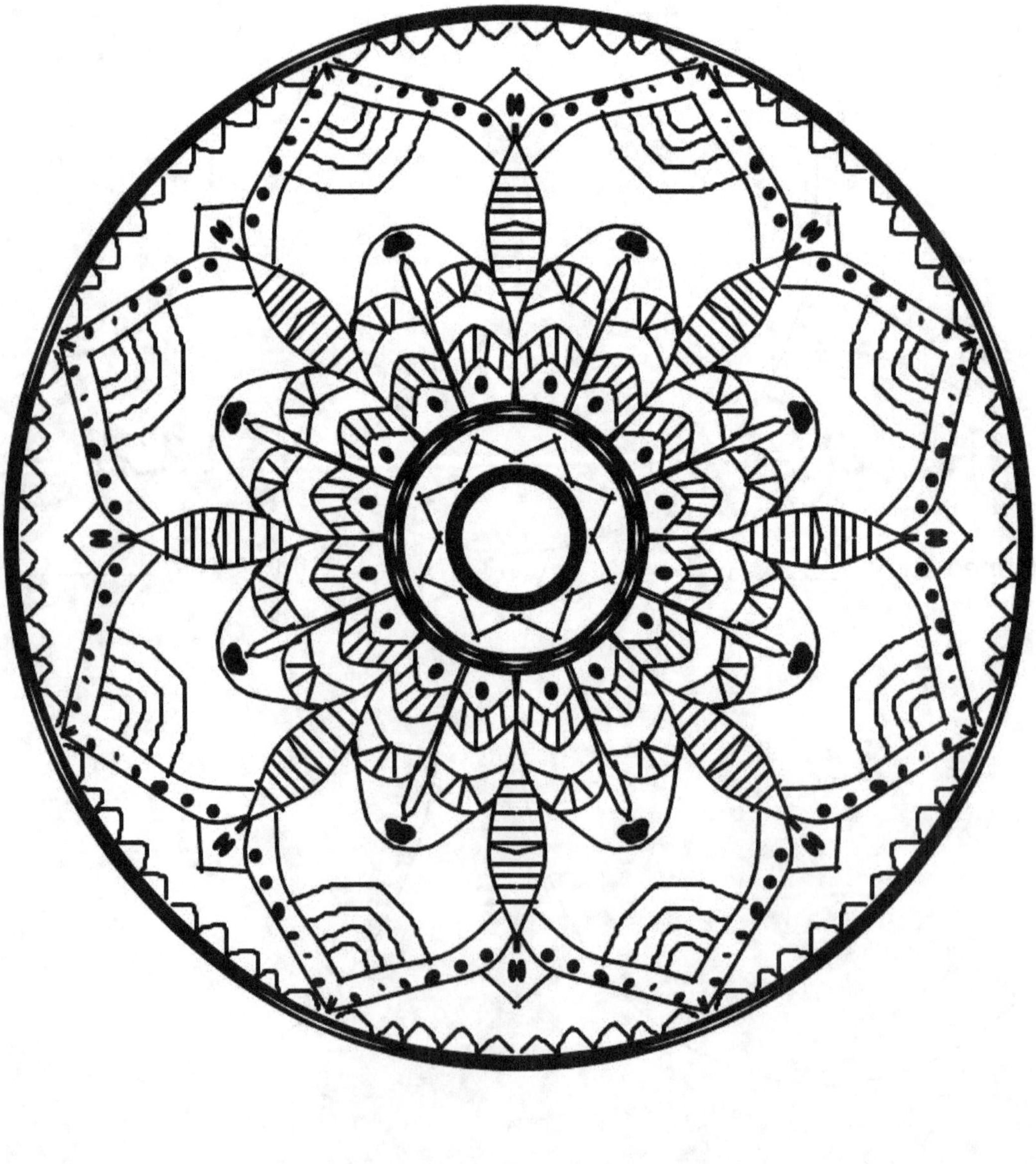

Day Twenty-five _______

5:00 _______________________

6:00 _______________________

7:00 _______________________

8:00 _______________________

9:00 _______________________

10:00 ______________________

11:00 ______________________

Noon _______________________

1:00 _______________________

2:00 _______________________

3:00 _______________________

4:00 _______________________

5:00 _______________________

6:00 _______________________

7:00 _______________________

8:00 _______________________

9:00 _______________________

10:00 ______________________

11:00 ______________________

Midnight ____________________

top priorities for today 🎯

____

____

____

____

Today's victories 🏆

Make it your mission to stay positive. Write your positive mission statement.

____

____

____

____

____

The Workout

Exercise	Set 1	Set 2	Set 3	Set 4	Set 5	notes

Time started: _____________   Time ended: _____________

Location: ____

Feelings before training:

Feelings after training

NUTRITION

Meal 1

time eaten: _________

Meal 2

time eaten: _________

Meal 3

time eaten: _________

Meal 4

time eaten: _________

Meal 5

time eaten: _________

Hydration

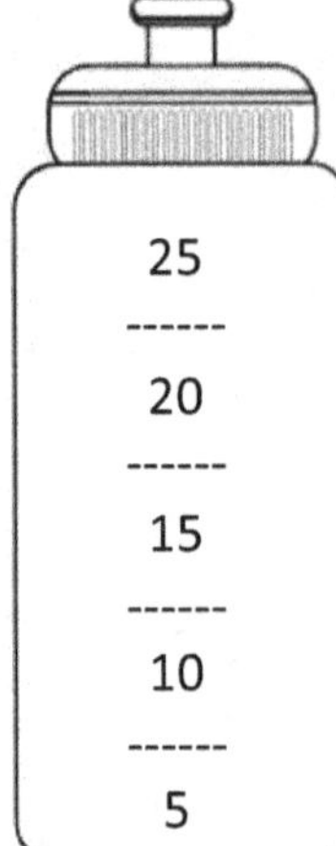

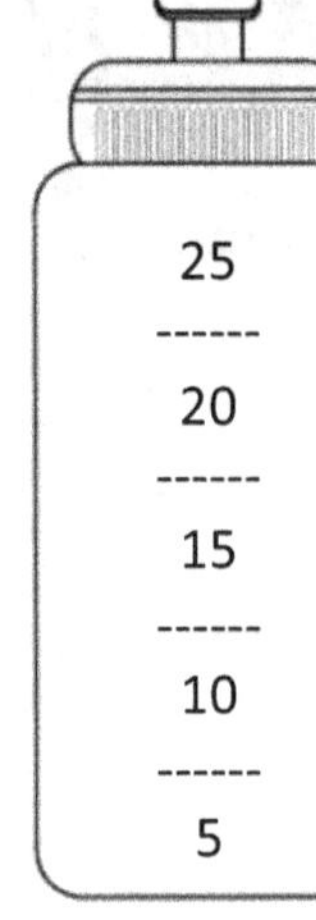

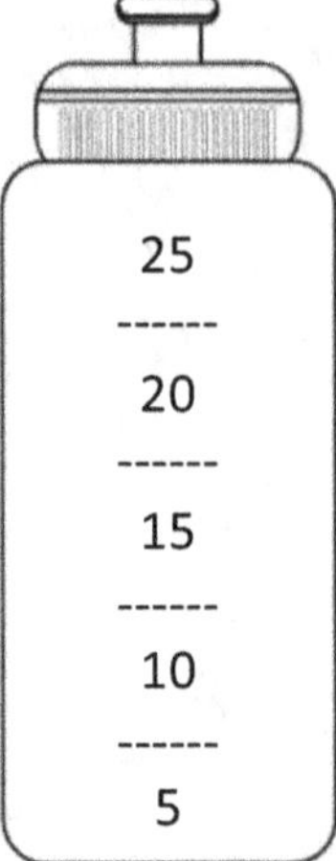

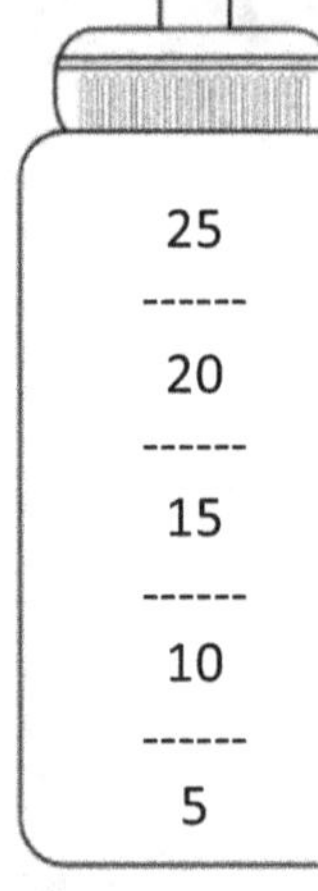

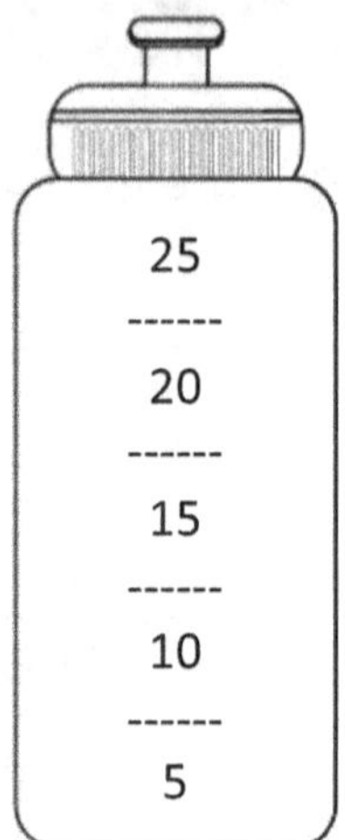

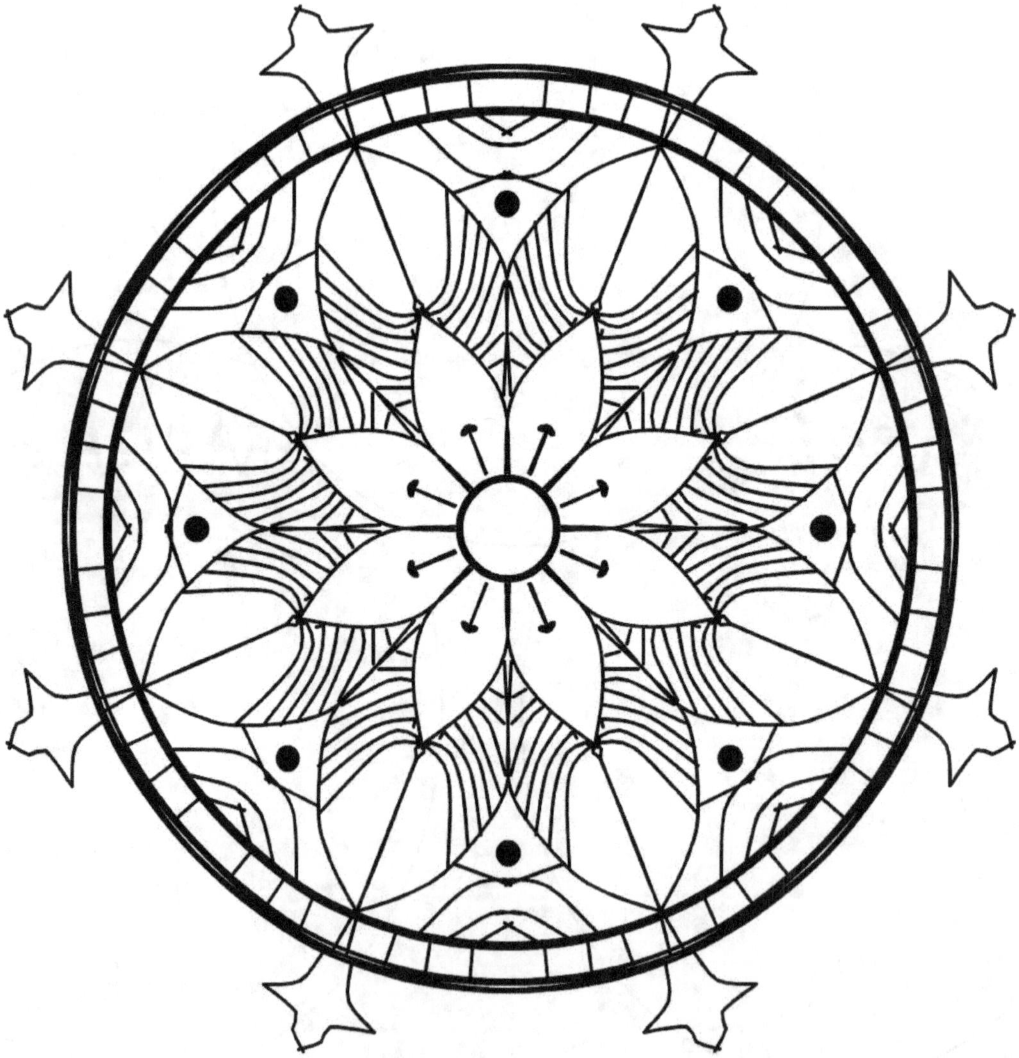

Day Twenty-six _______

5:00 ________________________

6:00 ________________________

7:00 ________________________

8:00 ________________________

9:00 ________________________

10:00 ________________________

11:00 ________________________

Noon ________________________

1:00 ________________________

2:00 ________________________

3:00 ________________________

4:00 ________________________

5:00 ________________________

6:00 ________________________

7:00 ________________________

8:00 ________________________

9:00 ________________________

10:00 ________________________

11:00 ________________________

Midnight ____________________

top priorities for today

Today's victories

What give you your inner energy?

The Stella Society Workout

Exercise	Set 1	Set 2	Set 3	Set 4	Set 5	notes

Time started: _____________   Time ended: _____________

Location: ____

Feelings before training:

Feelings after training

NUTRITION

Meal 1
time eaten: __________

Meal 2
time eaten: __________

Meal 3
time eaten: __________

Meal 4
time eaten: __________

Meal 5
time eaten: __________

Hydration

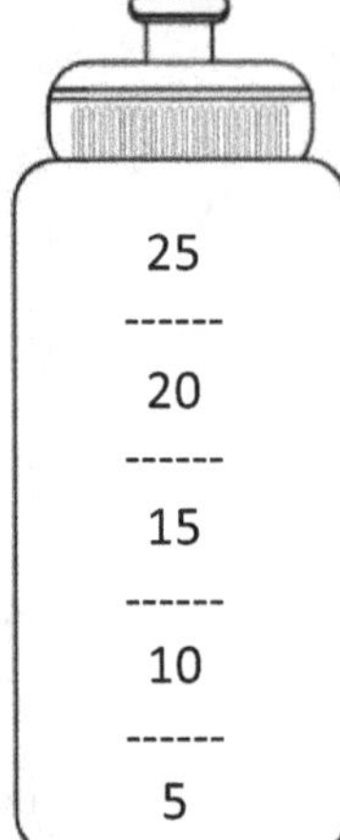

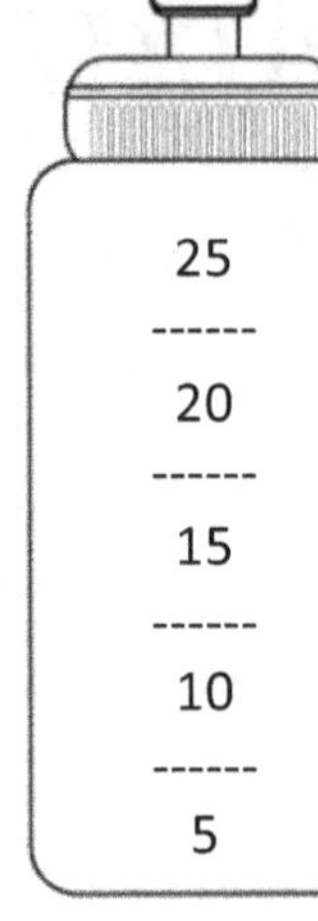

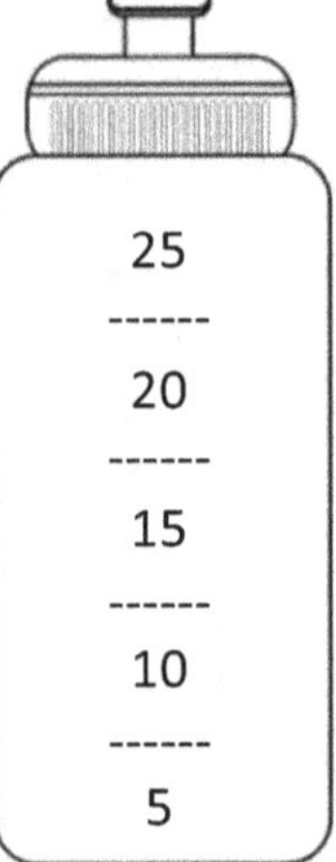

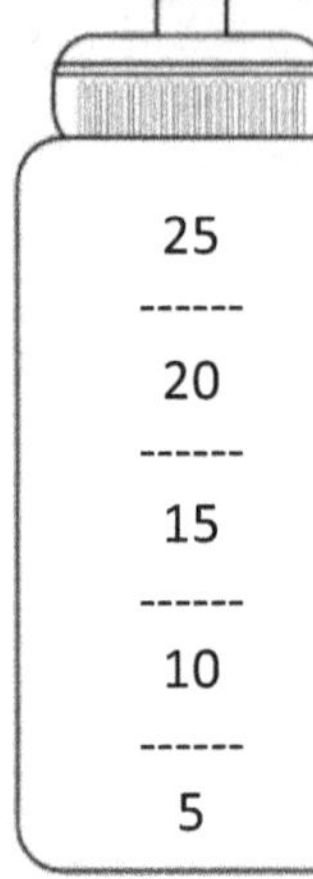

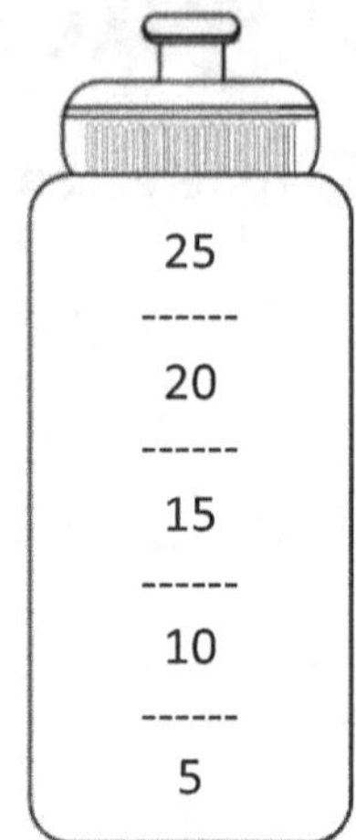

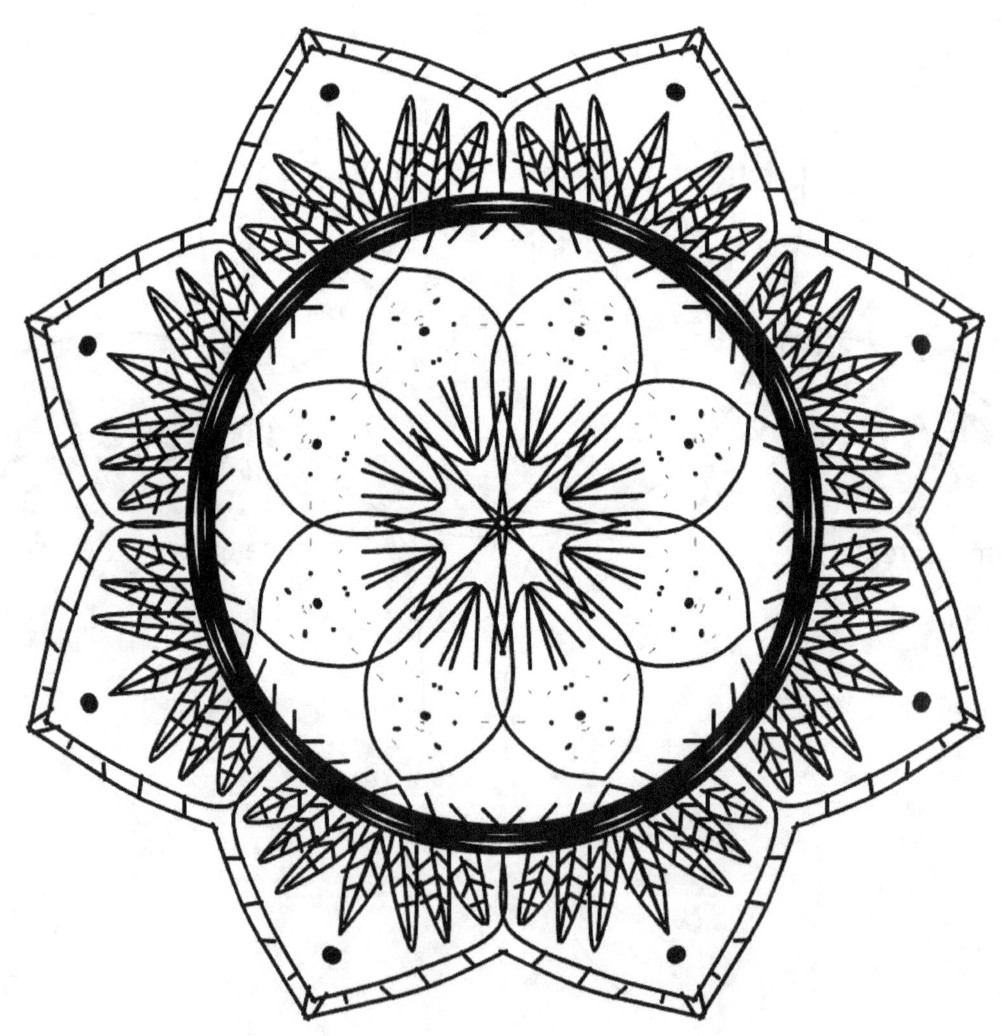

Day Twenty-seven _______

5:00 _______________________

6:00 _______________________

7:00 _______________________

8:00 _______________________

9:00 _______________________

10:00 ______________________

11:00 ______________________

Noon _______________________

1:00 _______________________

2:00 _______________________

3:00 _______________________

4:00 _______________________

5:00 _______________________

6:00 _______________________

7:00 _______________________

8:00 _______________________

9:00 _______________________

10:00 ______________________

11:00 ______________________

Midnight ___________________

top priorities for today 🎯

____

____

____

____

Today's victories 🏆

What have you stopped, but won't stop again?

____

____

____

____

____

____

The *Stella Society* Workout

Exercise	Set 1	Set 2	Set 3	Set 4	Set 5	notes

Time started: _____________ Time ended: _____________

Location: ____

Feelings before training:

Feelings after training

NUTRITION

Meal 1
time eaten: __________

Meal 2
time eaten: __________

Meal 3
time eaten: __________

Meal 4
time eaten: __________

Meal 5
time eaten: __________

Hydration

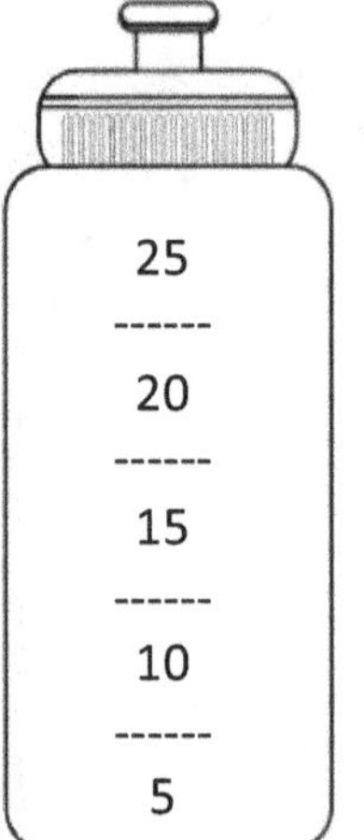

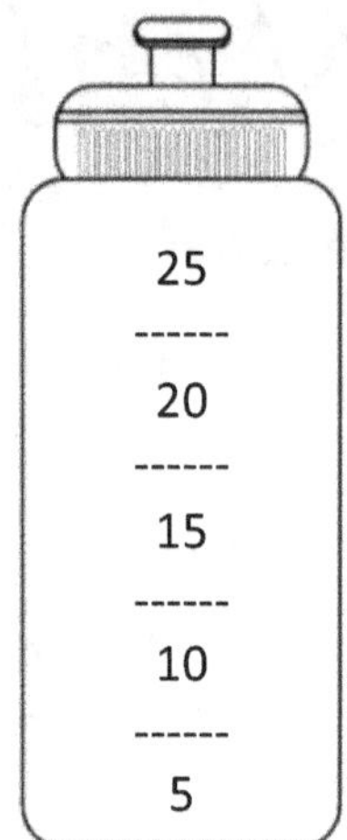

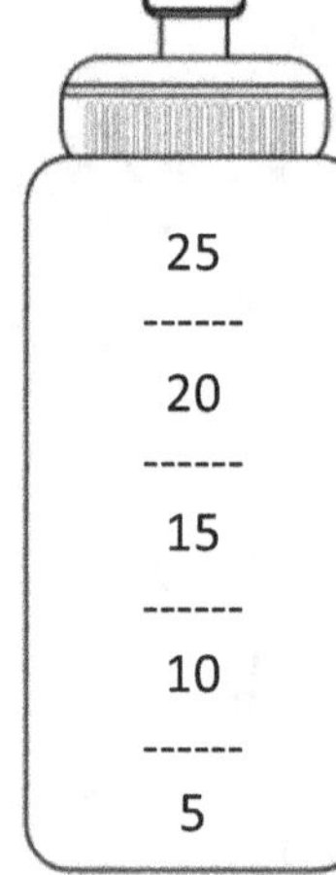

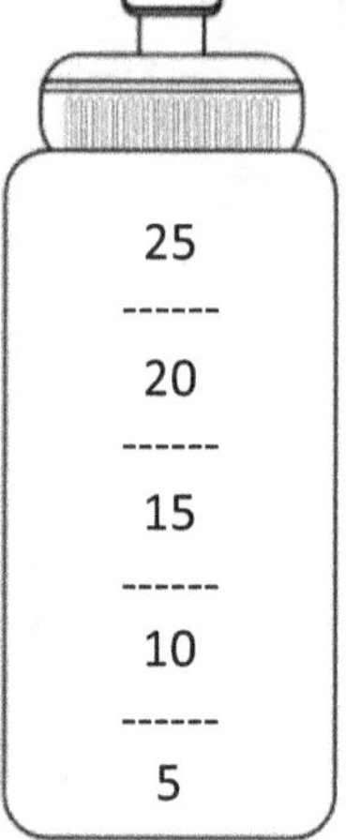

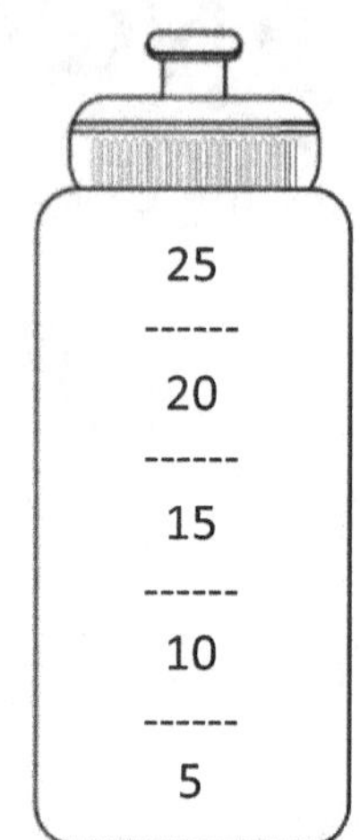

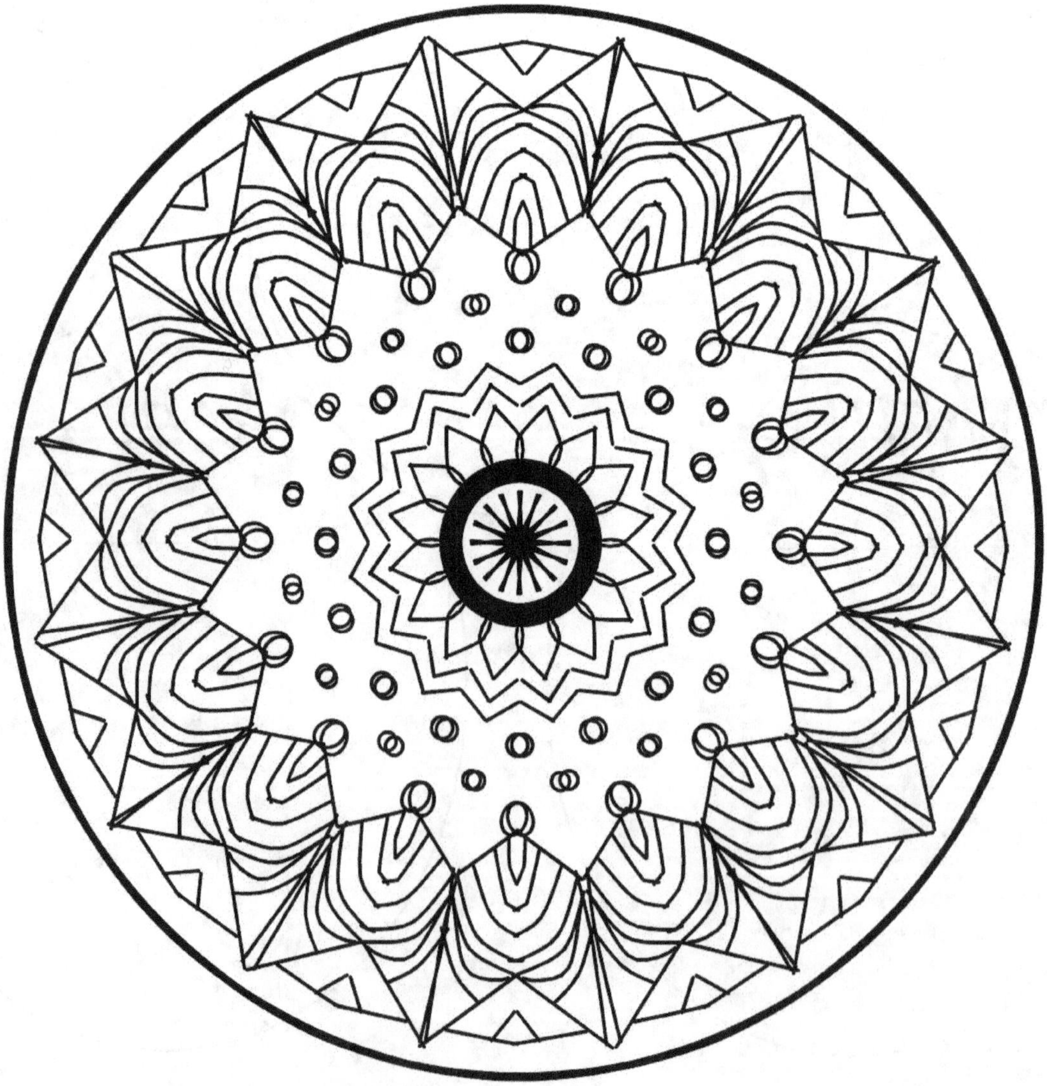

Day Twenty-eight ______

5:00 _______________	
6:00 _______________	
7:00 _______________	

top priorities for today 🎯

____

5:00 _____________________

6:00 _____________________

7:00 _____________________

8:00 _____________________

9:00 _____________________

10:00 _____________________

11:00 _____________________

Noon _____________________

1:00 _____________________

2:00 _____________________

3:00 _____________________

4:00 _____________________

5:00 _____________________

6:00 _____________________

7:00 _____________________

8:00 _____________________

9:00 _____________________

10:00 _____________________

11:00 _____________________

Midnight _____________________

Today's victories 🏆

How do identify with being
a unicorn?

____

____

____

____

____

The Stella Society Workout

Exercise	Set 1	Set 2	Set 3	Set 4	Set 5	notes

Time started: _______________   Time ended: _______________

Location: ____

Feelings before training: 🙂 😐 🙁 😜 😣 😔 😇 😎

Feelings after training 🙂 😐 🙁 😜 😣 😔 😇 😎

NUTRITION

Meal 1
time eaten: __________

Meal 2
time eaten: __________

Meal 3
time eaten: __________

Meal 4
time eaten: __________

Meal 5
time eaten: __________

Hydration

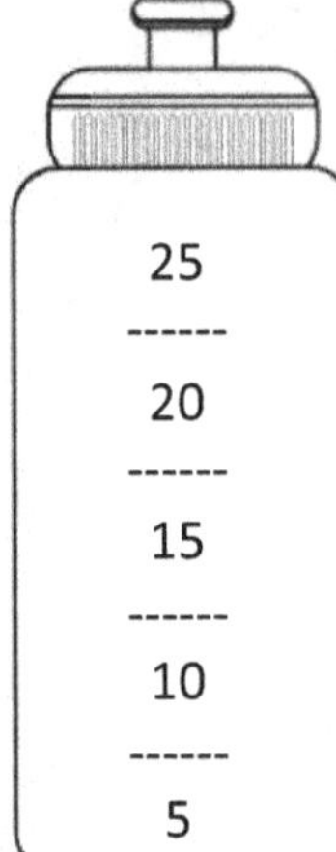

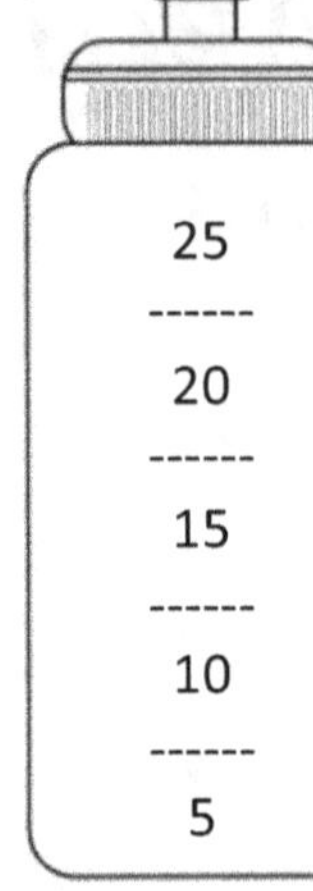

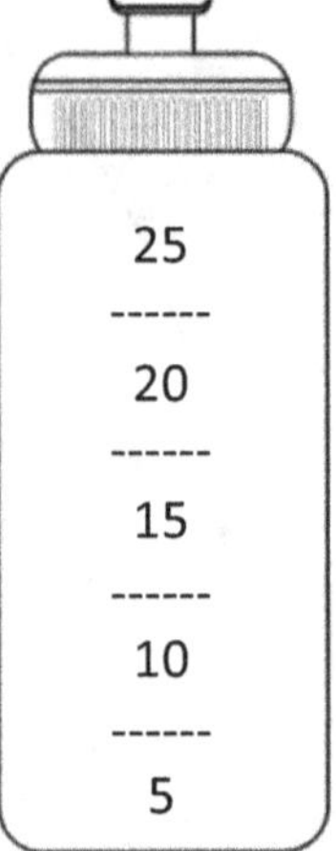

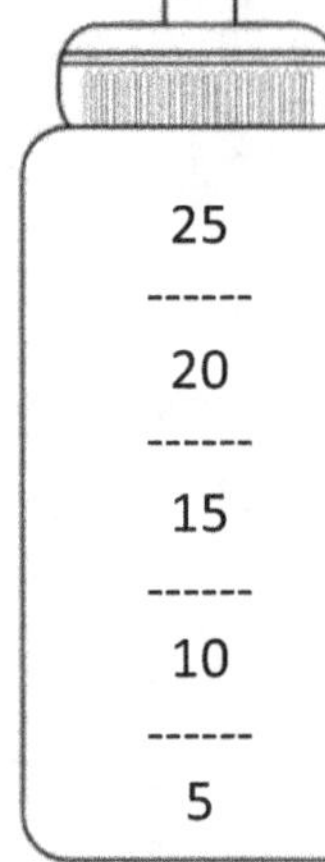

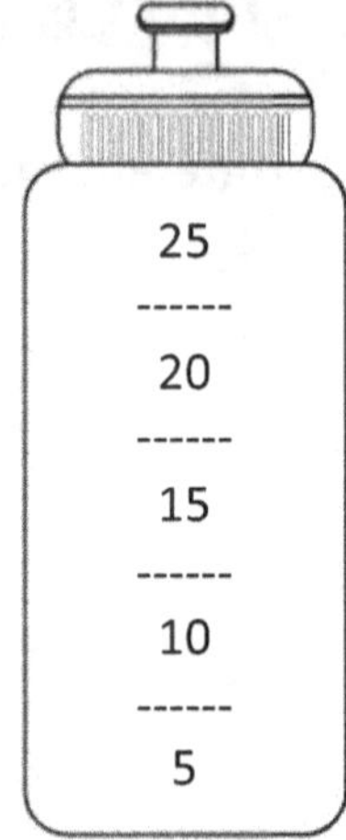

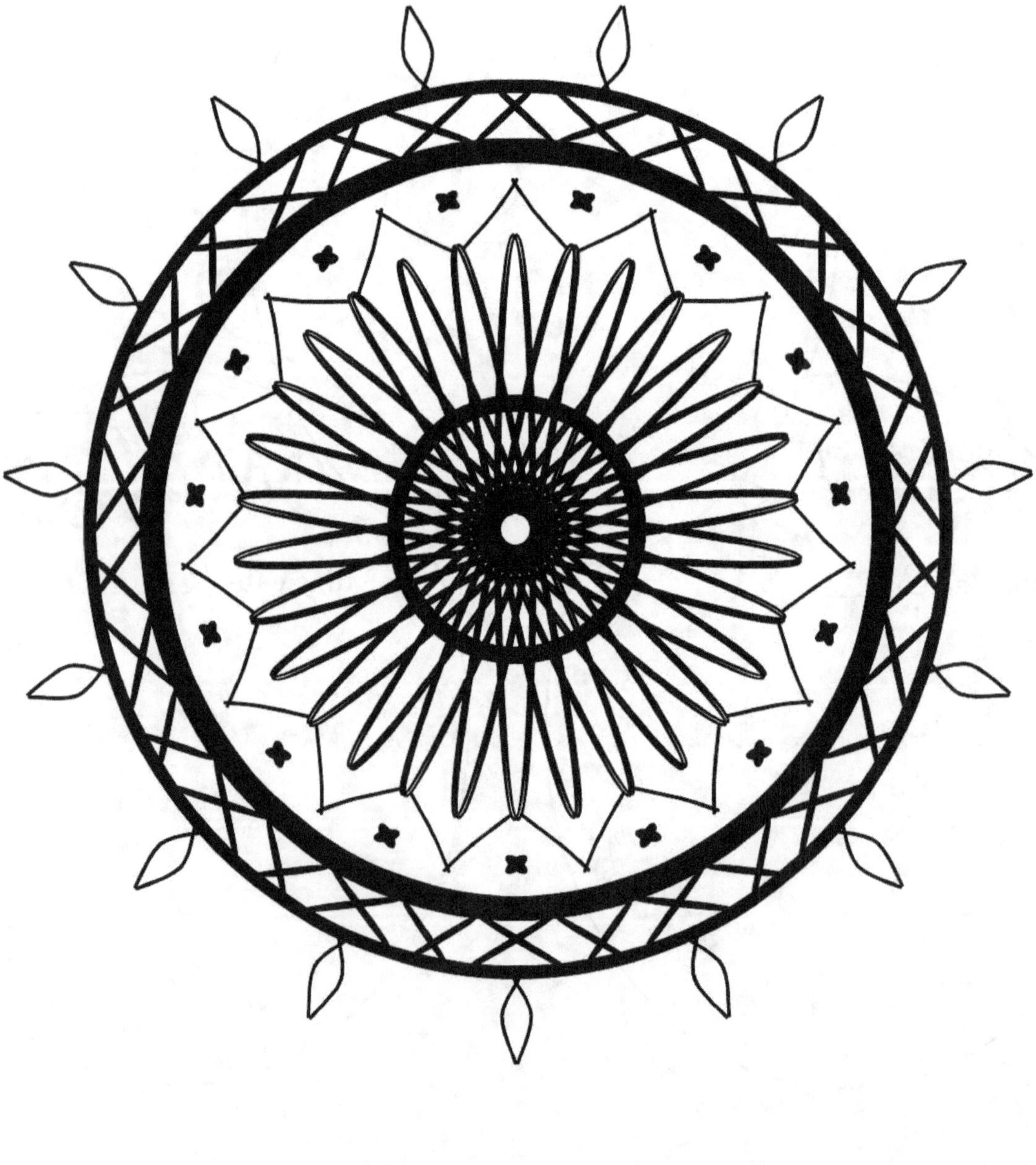

Day Twenty-nine _______

5:00 _______________________

6:00 _______________________

7:00 _______________________

8:00 _______________________

9:00 _______________________

10:00 ______________________

11:00 ______________________

Noon _______________________

1:00 _______________________

2:00 _______________________

3:00 _______________________

4:00 _______________________

5:00 _______________________

6:00 _______________________

7:00 _______________________

8:00 _______________________

9:00 _______________________

10:00 ______________________

11:00 ______________________

Midnight ___________________

____

____

____

____

You have permission to be a
savage. What do you do with it?

____

____

____

____

____

The *Stella Society* Workout

Exercise	Set 1	Set 2	Set 3	Set 4	Set 5	notes

Time started: _____________   Time ended: _____________

Location: ____

Feelings before training:

Feelings after training

NUTRITION

Meal 1
time eaten: _________

Meal 2
time eaten: _________

Meal 3
time eaten: _________

Meal 4
time eaten: _________

Meal 5
time eaten: _________

Hydration

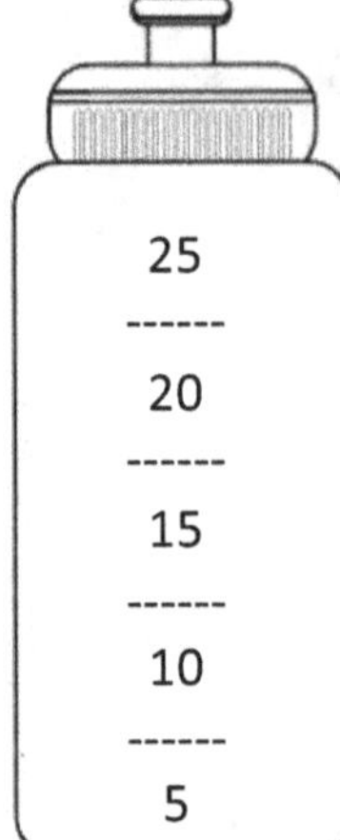

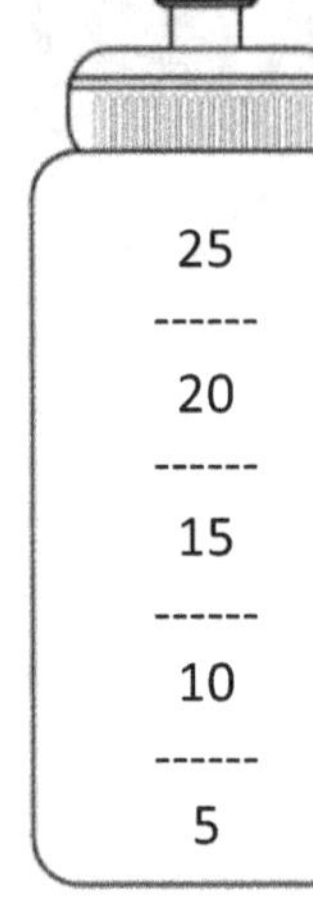

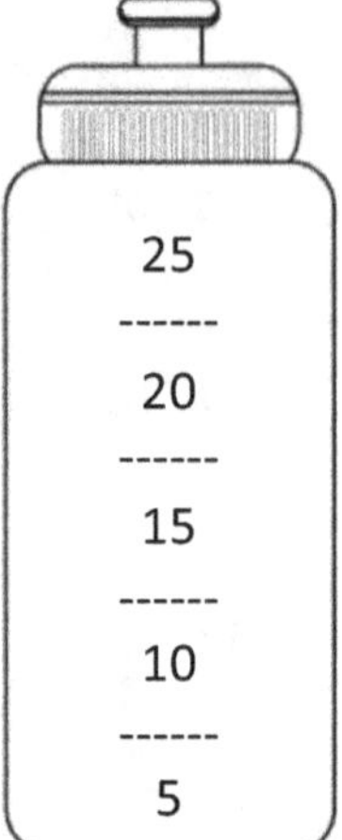

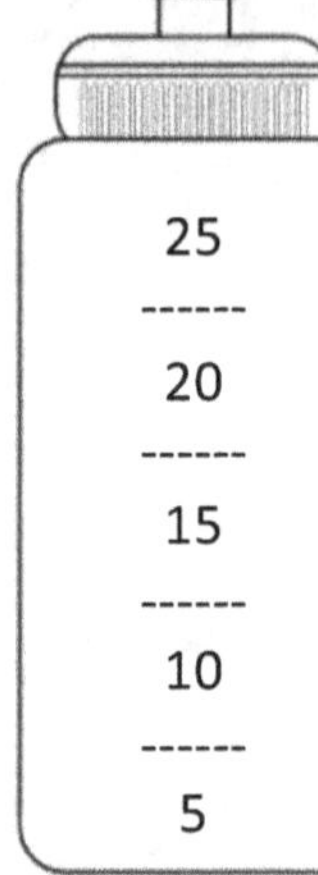

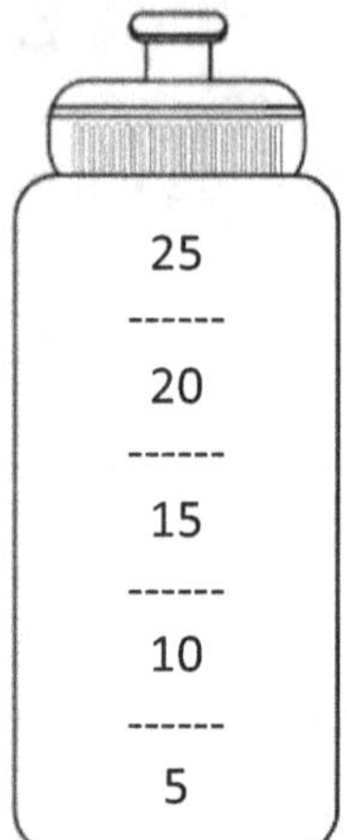

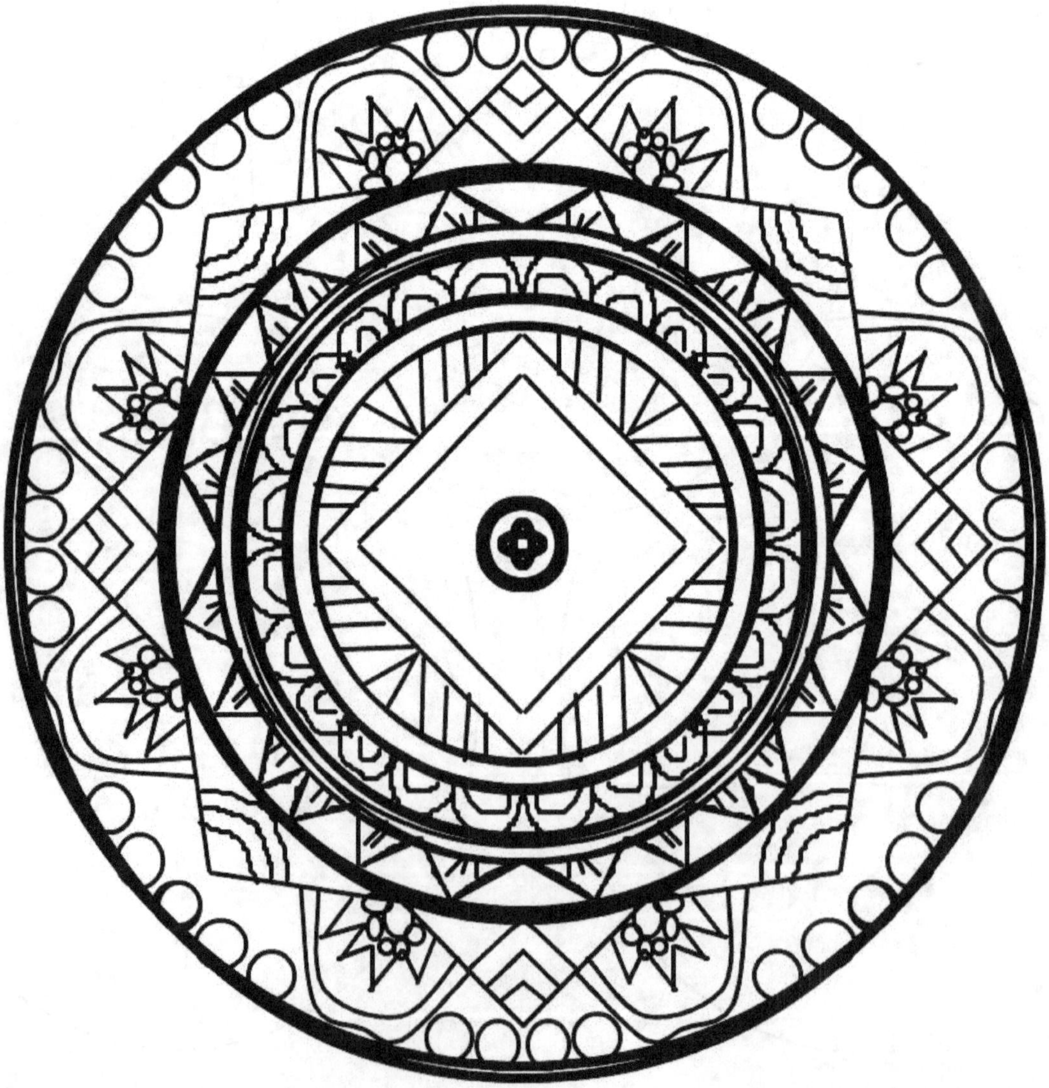

Measurements

DATE: ___________

Weight: _______

Neck _______

Shoulders _______

Chest _______

Bicep / upper arm left _________ right _________

Forearm left _________ right _______

Waist _______

Hips _______

Thighs left _________ right _______

Calf left _________ right _______

It's Not A Diet,
It's A Lifestyle Change

Day Thirty ______

Time	
5:00	_________________
6:00	_________________
7:00	_________________
8:00	_________________
9:00	_________________
10:00	_________________
11:00	_________________
Noon	_________________
1:00	_________________
2:00	_________________
3:00	_________________
4:00	_________________
5:00	_________________
6:00	_________________
7:00	_________________
8:00	_________________
9:00	_________________
10:00	_________________
11:00	_________________
Midnight	_________________

How can you be powerful and sensitive at the same time?

The 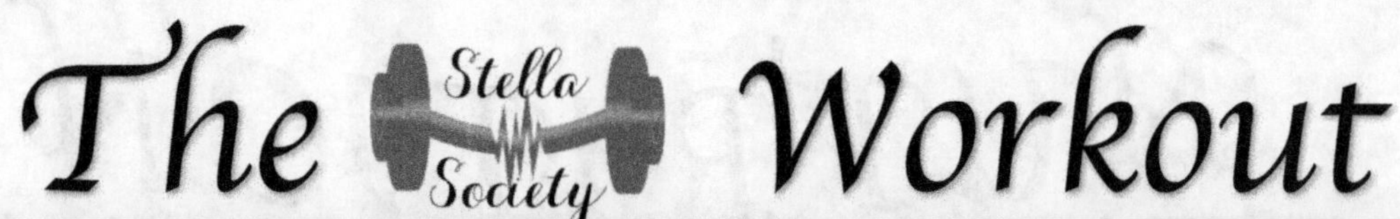 Workout

Exercise	Set 1	Set 2	Set 3	Set 4	Set 5	notes

Time started: _____________ Time ended: _____________

Location: ____

Feelings before training:        

Feelings after training

NUTRITION

Meal 1

time eaten: _________

Meal 2

time eaten: _________

Meal 3

time eaten: _________

Meal 4

time eaten: _________

Meal 5

time eaten: _________

Hydration

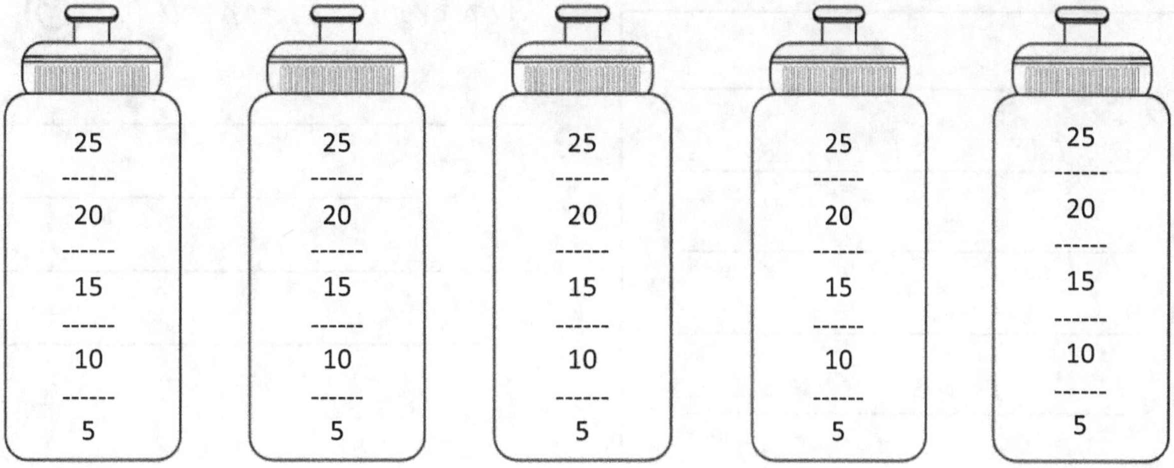

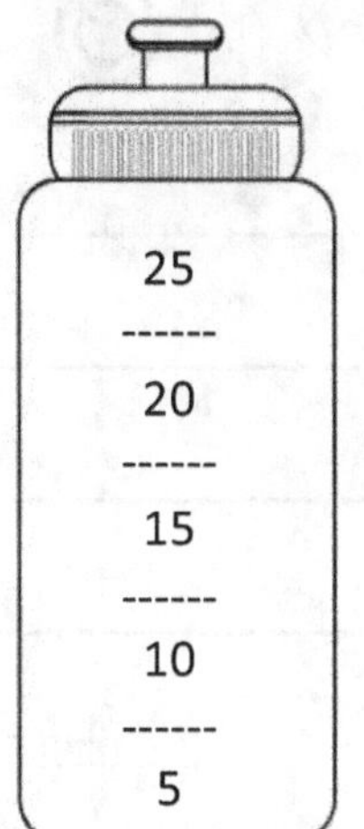
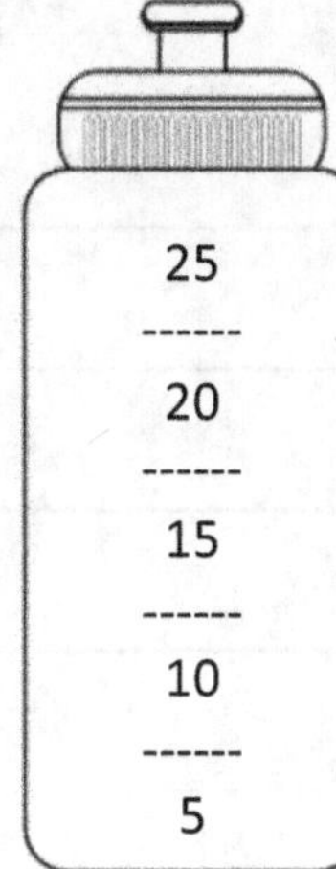
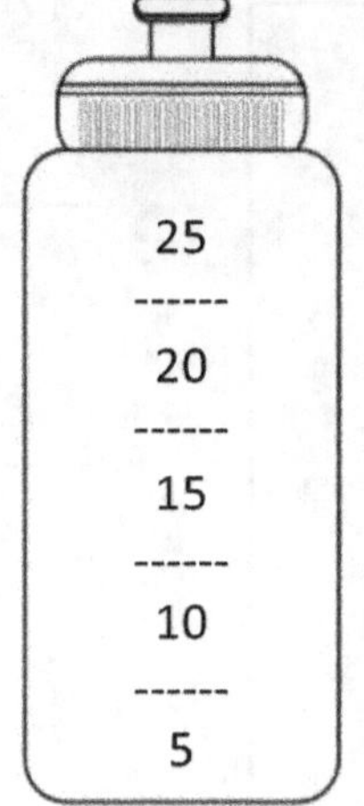
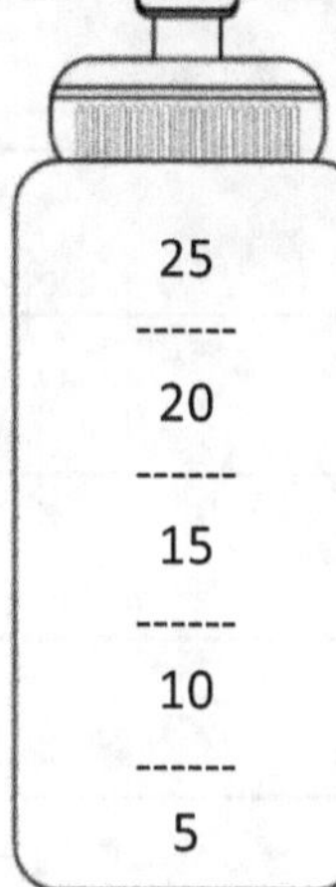
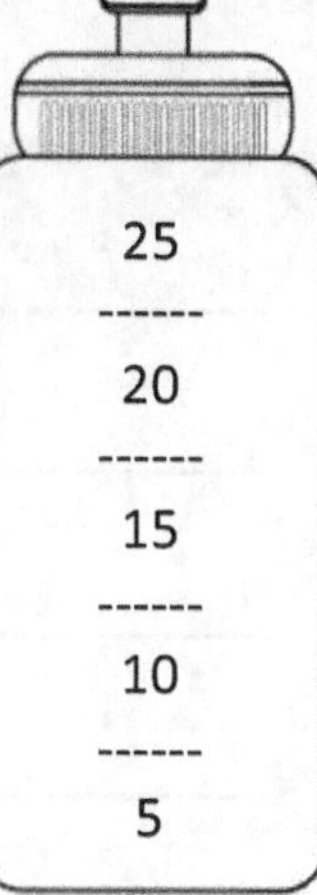

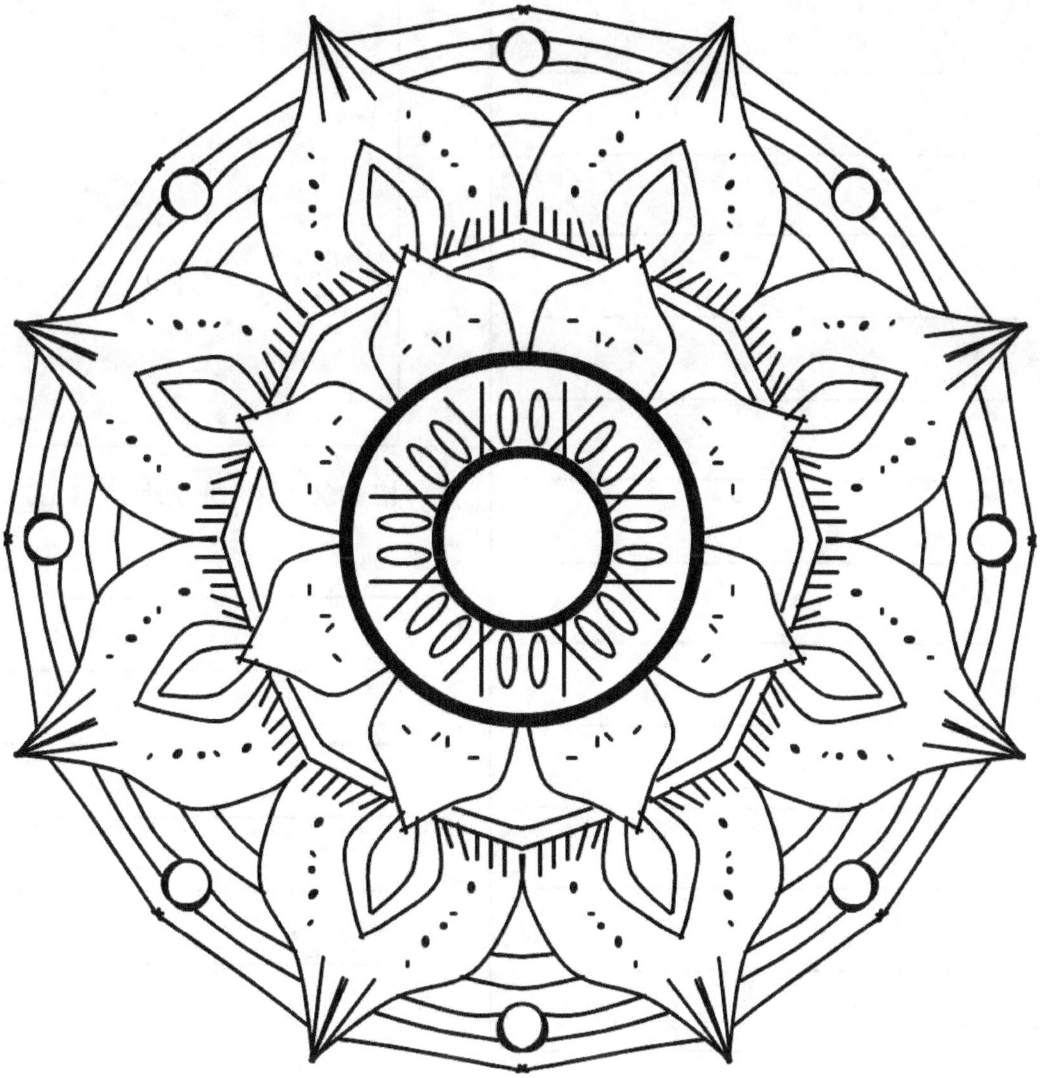

Day Thirty-one ______

5:00	_______________
6:00	_______________
7:00	_______________
8:00	_______________
9:00	_______________
10:00	_______________
11:00	_______________
Noon	_______________
1:00	_______________
2:00	_______________
3:00	_______________
4:00	_______________
5:00	_______________
6:00	_______________
7:00	_______________
8:00	_______________
9:00	_______________
10:00	_______________
11:00	_______________
Midnight	_______________

Today's victories

Is being forceful a bad thing?

The 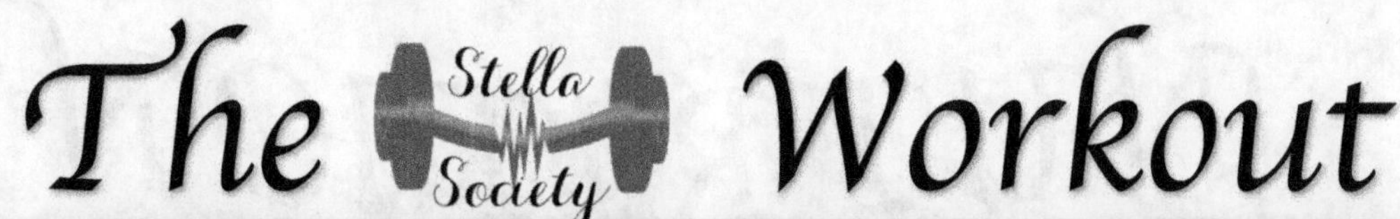 Workout

Exercise	Set 1	Set 2	Set 3	Set 4	Set 5	notes

Time started: _____________ Time ended: _____________

Location: ____

Feelings before training: 🙂 😐 ☹️ 😜 😣 😟 😊 😎

Feelings after training 🙂 😐 ☹️ 😜 😣 😟 😊 😎

NUTRITION

Meal 1

time eaten: _________

Meal 2

time eaten: _________

Meal 3

time eaten: _________

Meal 4

time eaten: _________

Meal 5

time eaten: _________

Hydration

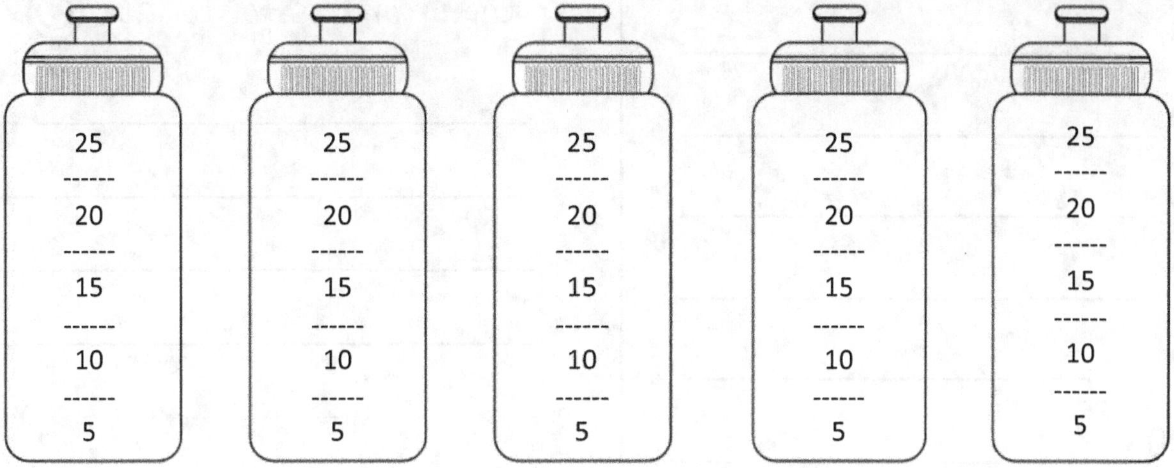

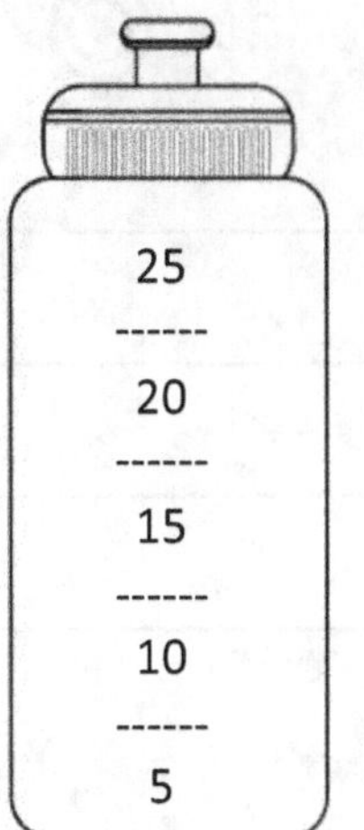 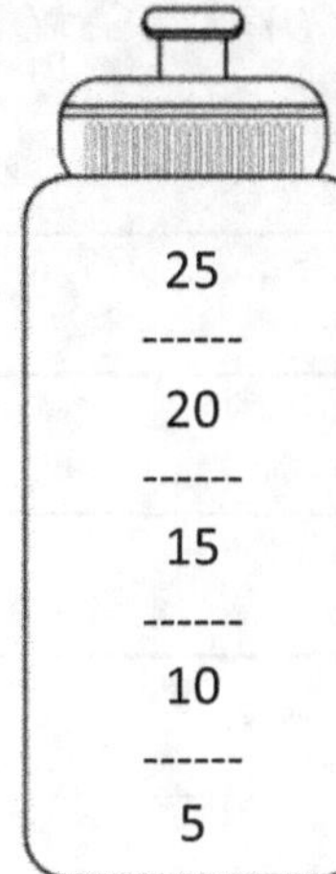

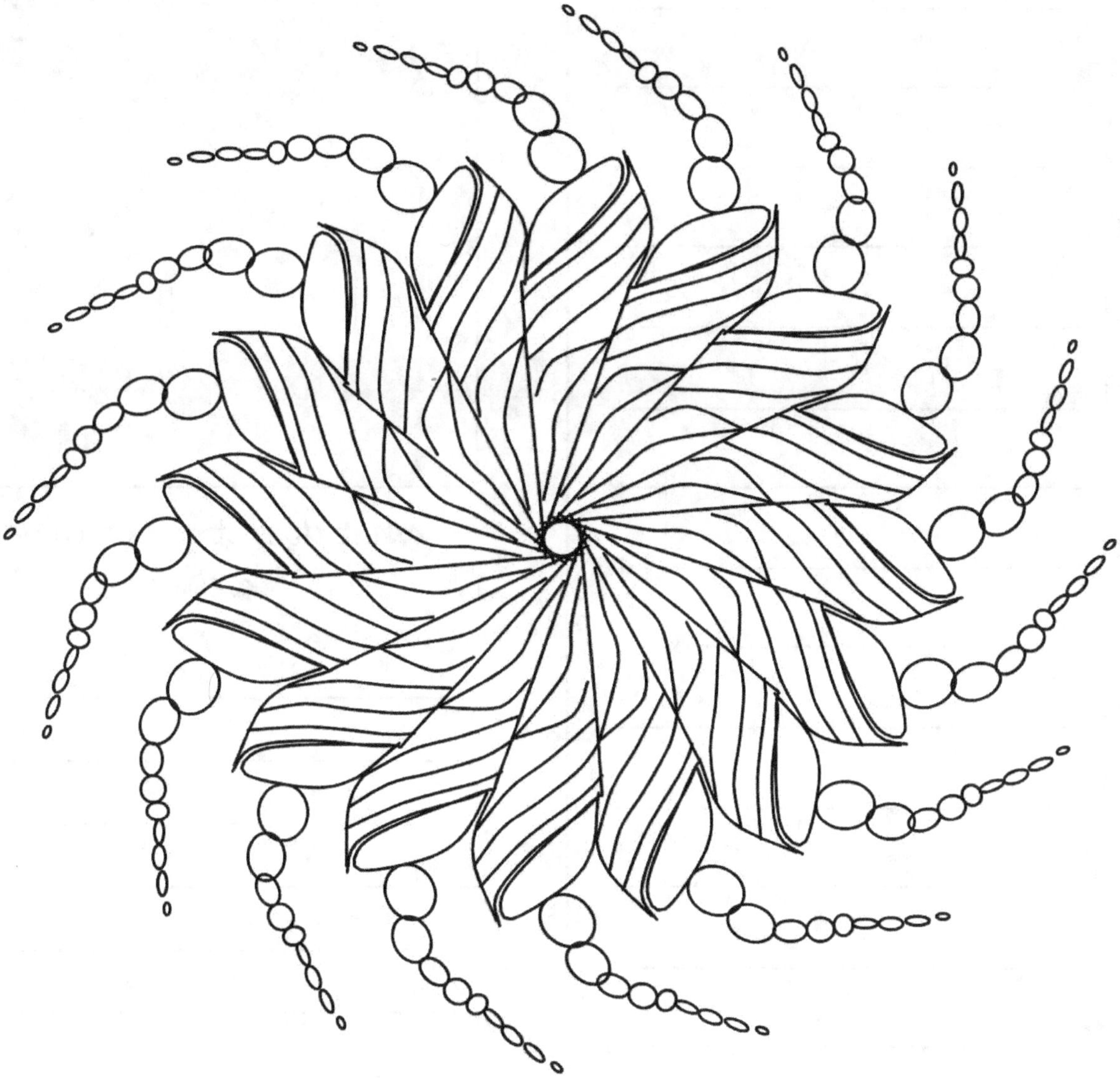

Day Thirty-two _______

<table>
<tr><td>

5:00 _______________________

6:00 _______________________

7:00 _______________________

8:00 _______________________

9:00 _______________________

10:00 ______________________

11:00 ______________________

Noon _______________________

1:00 _______________________

2:00 _______________________

3:00 _______________________

4:00 _______________________

5:00 _______________________

6:00 _______________________

7:00 _______________________

8:00 _______________________

9:00 _______________________

10:00 ______________________

11:00 ______________________

Midnight ___________________

</td><td>

top priorities for today 🎯

____

____

____

____

Today's victories 🏆

What does it mean to be fervent?

____

____

____

____

____

____

</td></tr>
</table>

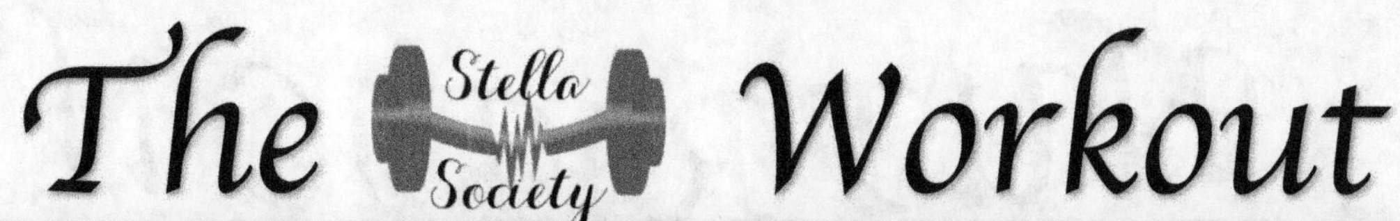

The Stella Society Workout

Exercise	Set 1	Set 2	Set 3	Set 4	Set 5	notes

Time started: _____________   Time ended: _____________

Location: ____

Feelings before training: 🙂 😐 ☹️ 😜 😠 😟 😊 😎

Feelings after training 🙂 😐 ☹️ 😜 😠 😟 😊 😎

NUTRITION

Meal 1

time eaten: _________

Meal 2

time eaten: _________

Meal 3

time eaten: _________

Meal 4

time eaten: _________

Meal 5

time eaten: _________

Hydration

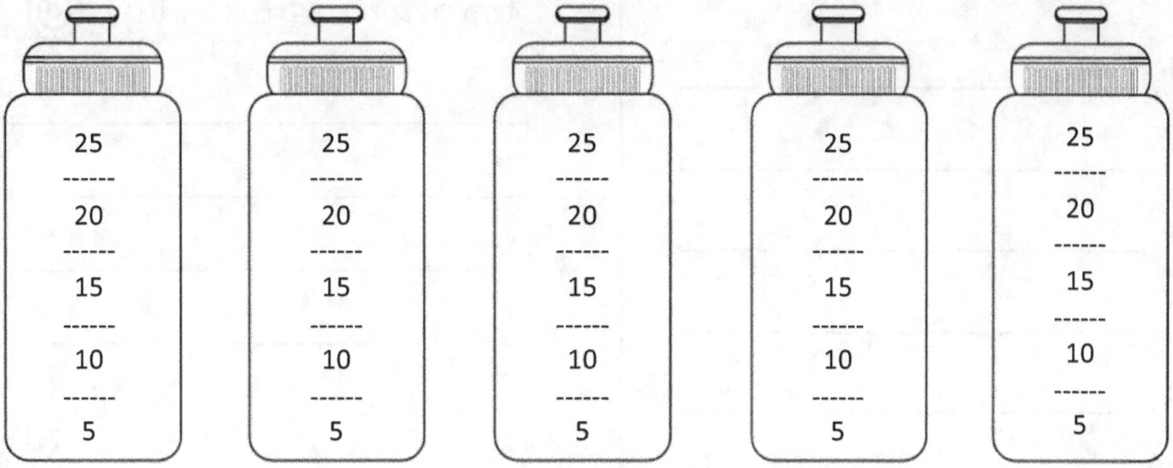

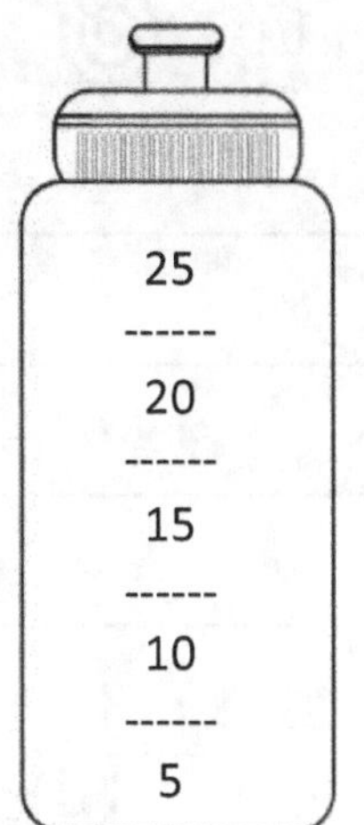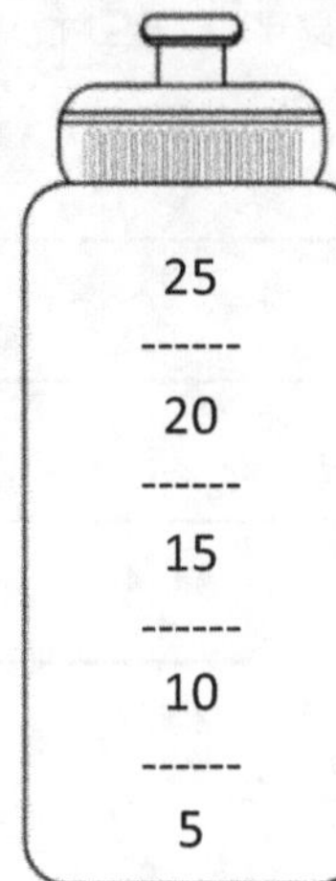

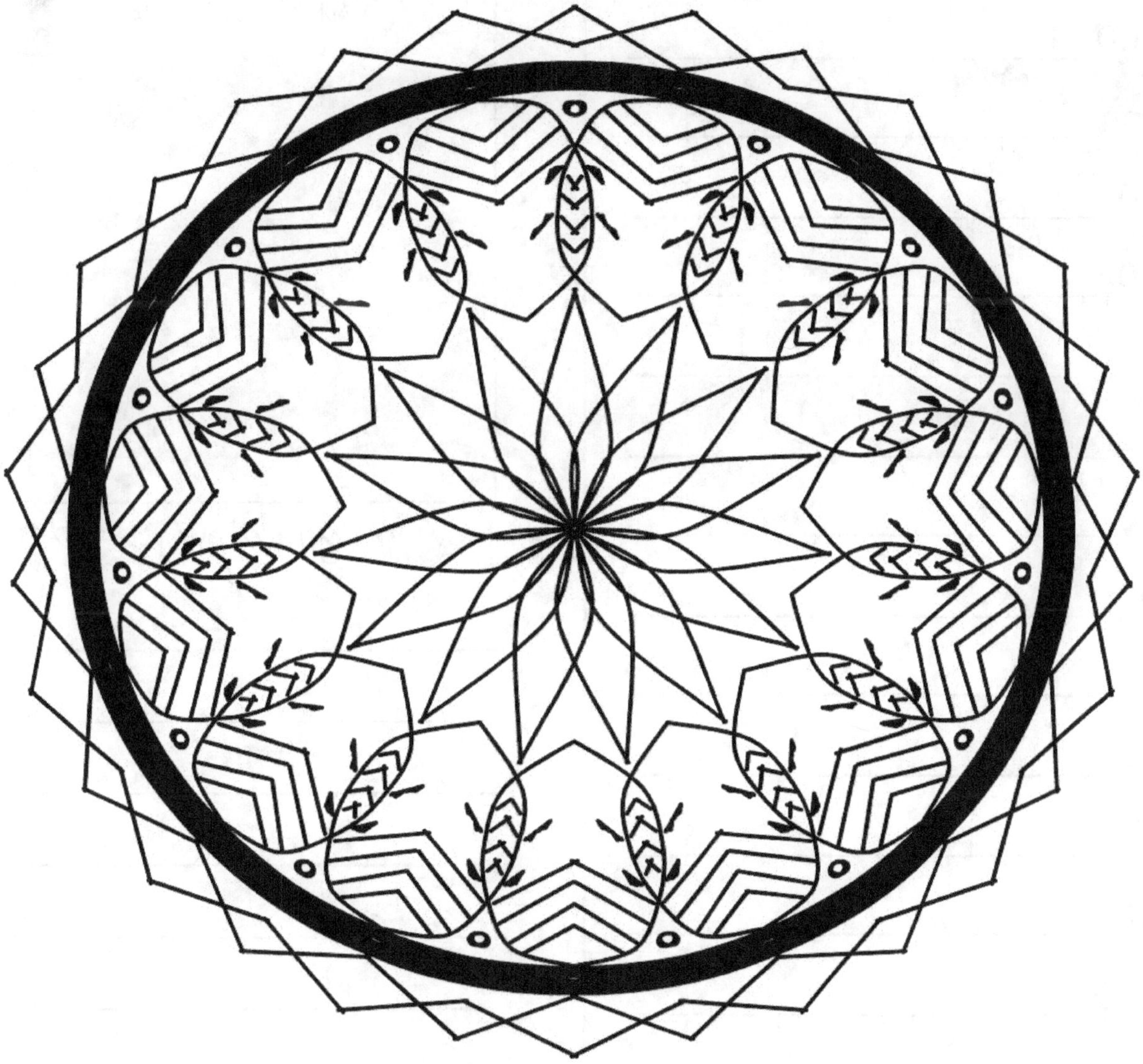

Day Thirty-three _______

5:00 _______________	

5:00 _______________

6:00 _______________

7:00 _______________

8:00 _______________

9:00 _______________

10:00 _______________

11:00 _______________

Noon _______________

1:00 _______________

2:00 _______________

3:00 _______________

4:00 _______________

5:00 _______________

6:00 _______________

7:00 _______________

8:00 _______________

9:00 _______________

10:00 _______________

11:00 _______________

Midnight _______________

top priorities for today

____
____
____
____

Today's victories

How are you glowing today?

____
____
____
____
____
____

The 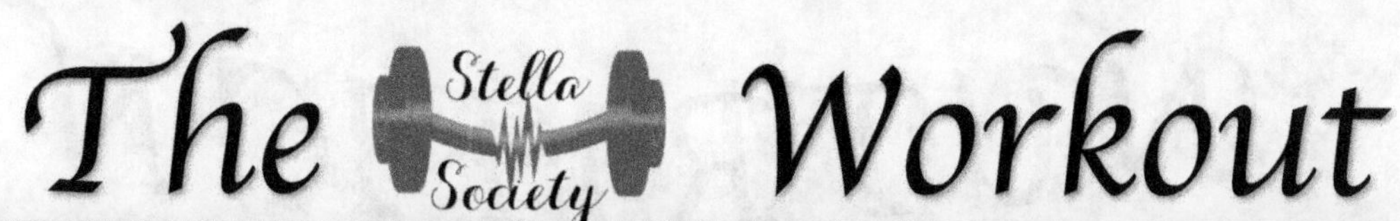 Workout

Exercise	Set 1	Set 2	Set 3	Set 4	Set 5	notes

Time started: _____________   Time ended: _____________

Location: ____

Feelings before training: 😊 😐 ☹️ 😜 😠 😕 😊 😎

Feelings after training 😊 😐 ☹️ 😜 😠 😕 😊 😎

NUTRITION

Meal 1

time eaten: _________

Meal 2

time eaten: _________

Meal 3

time eaten: _________

Meal 4

time eaten: _________

Meal 5

time eaten: _________

Hydration

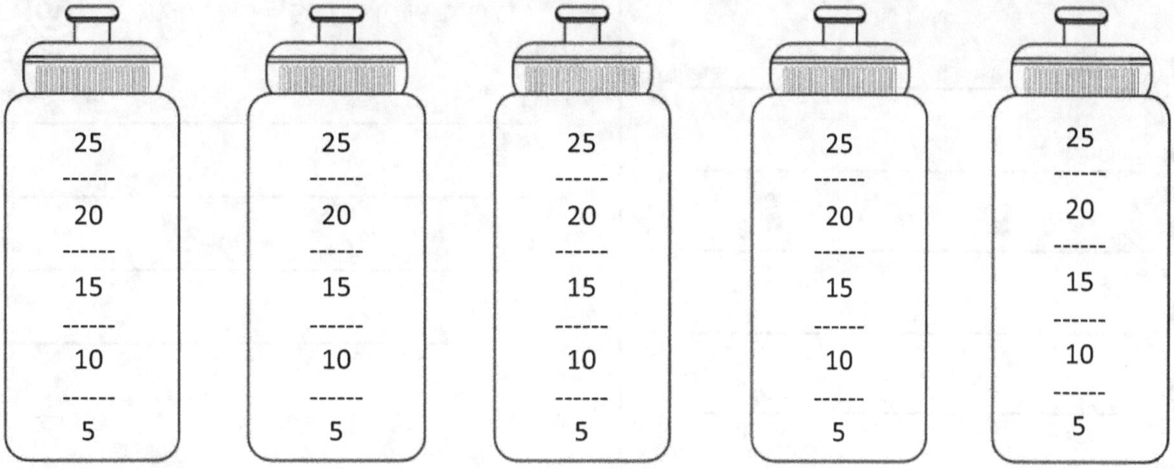

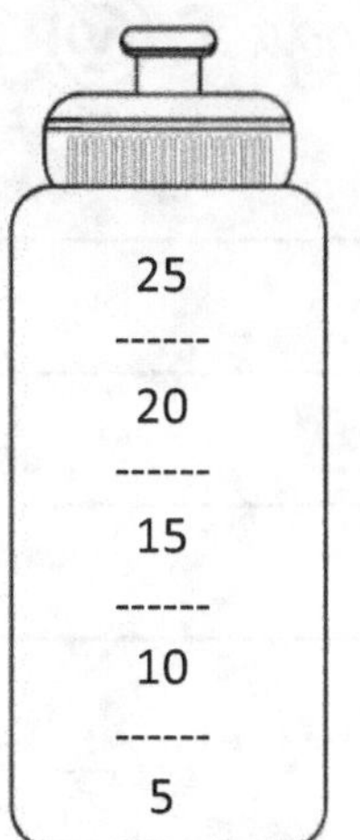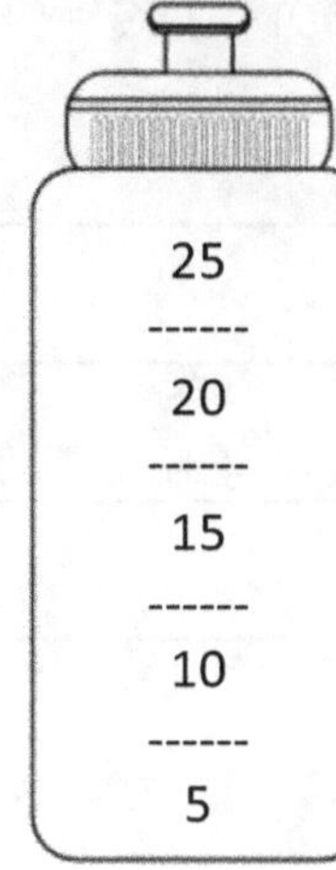

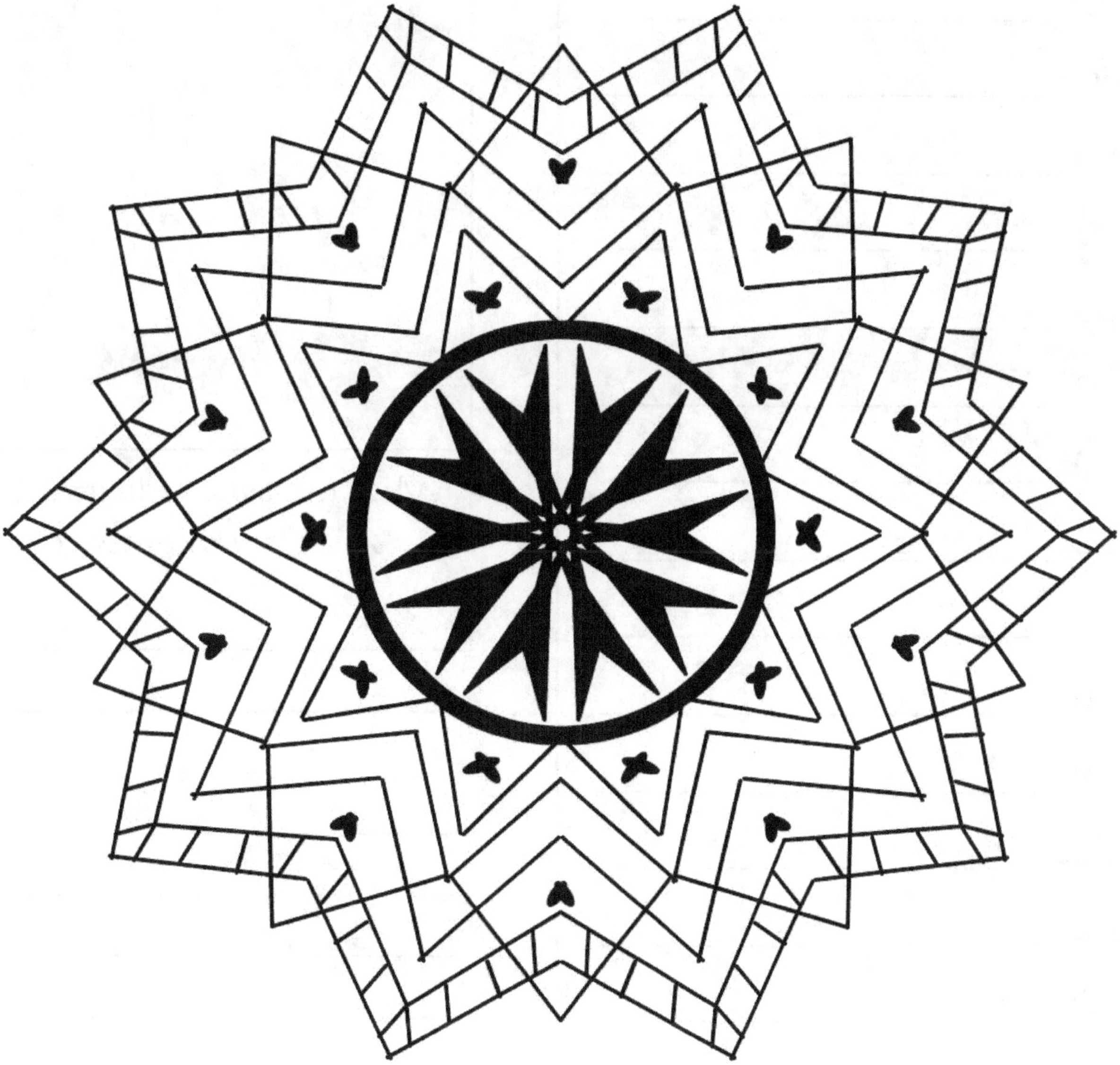

Day Thirty-four _______

5:00 _______________________

6:00 _______________________

7:00 _______________________

8:00 _______________________

9:00 _______________________

10:00 ______________________

11:00 ______________________

Noon _______________________

1:00 _______________________

2:00 _______________________

3:00 _______________________

4:00 _______________________

5:00 _______________________

6:00 _______________________

7:00 _______________________

8:00 _______________________

9:00 _______________________

10:00 ______________________

11:00 ______________________

Midnight ___________________

____

____

____

____

What are you dedicated to
do at this moment?

____

____

____

____

____

____

The Stella Society Workout

Exercise	Set 1	Set 2	Set 3	Set 4	Set 5	notes

Time started: _____________ Time ended: _____________

Location: _______________________________________

Feelings before training: 😊 😐 ☹ 😜 😠 😟 😇 😎

Feelings after training 😊 😐 ☹ 😜 😠 😟 😇 😎

NUTRITION

Meal 1

time eaten: _________

Meal 2

time eaten: _________

Meal 3

time eaten: _________

Meal 4

time eaten: _________

Meal 5

time eaten: _________

Hydration

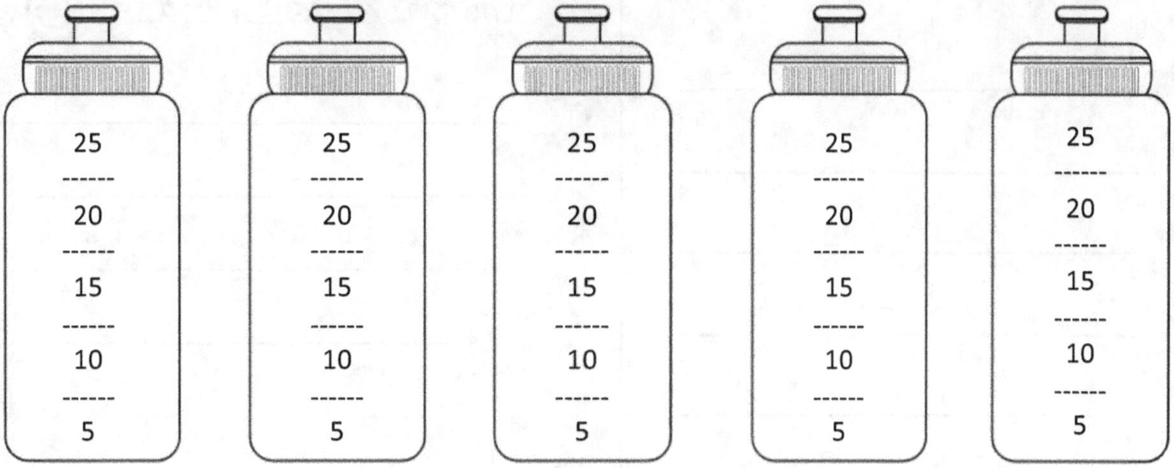

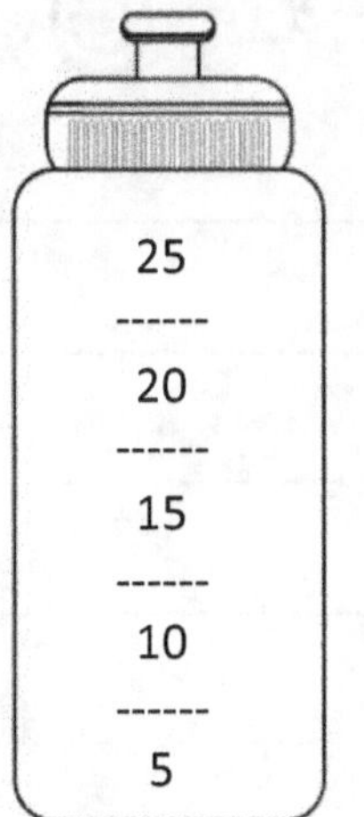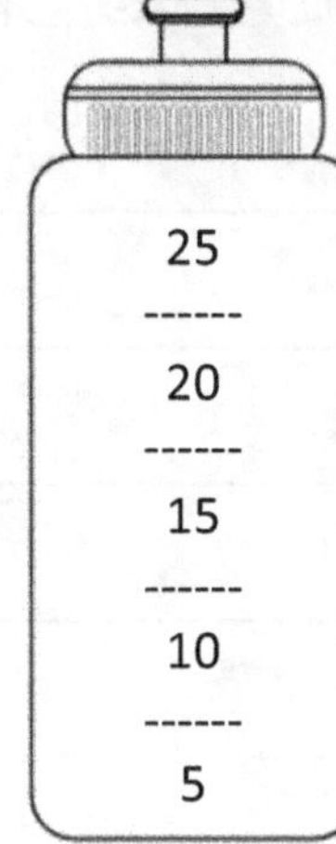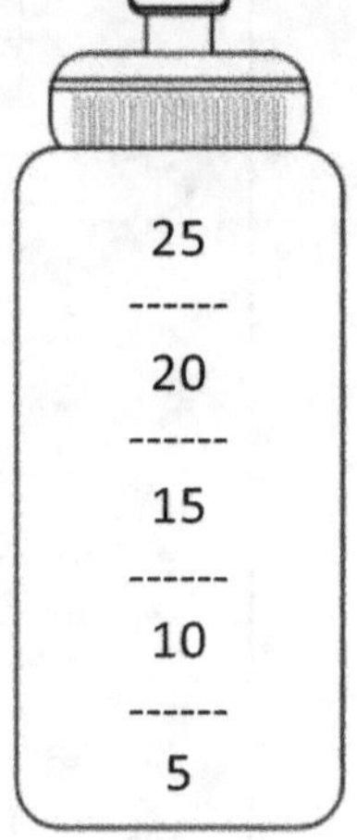

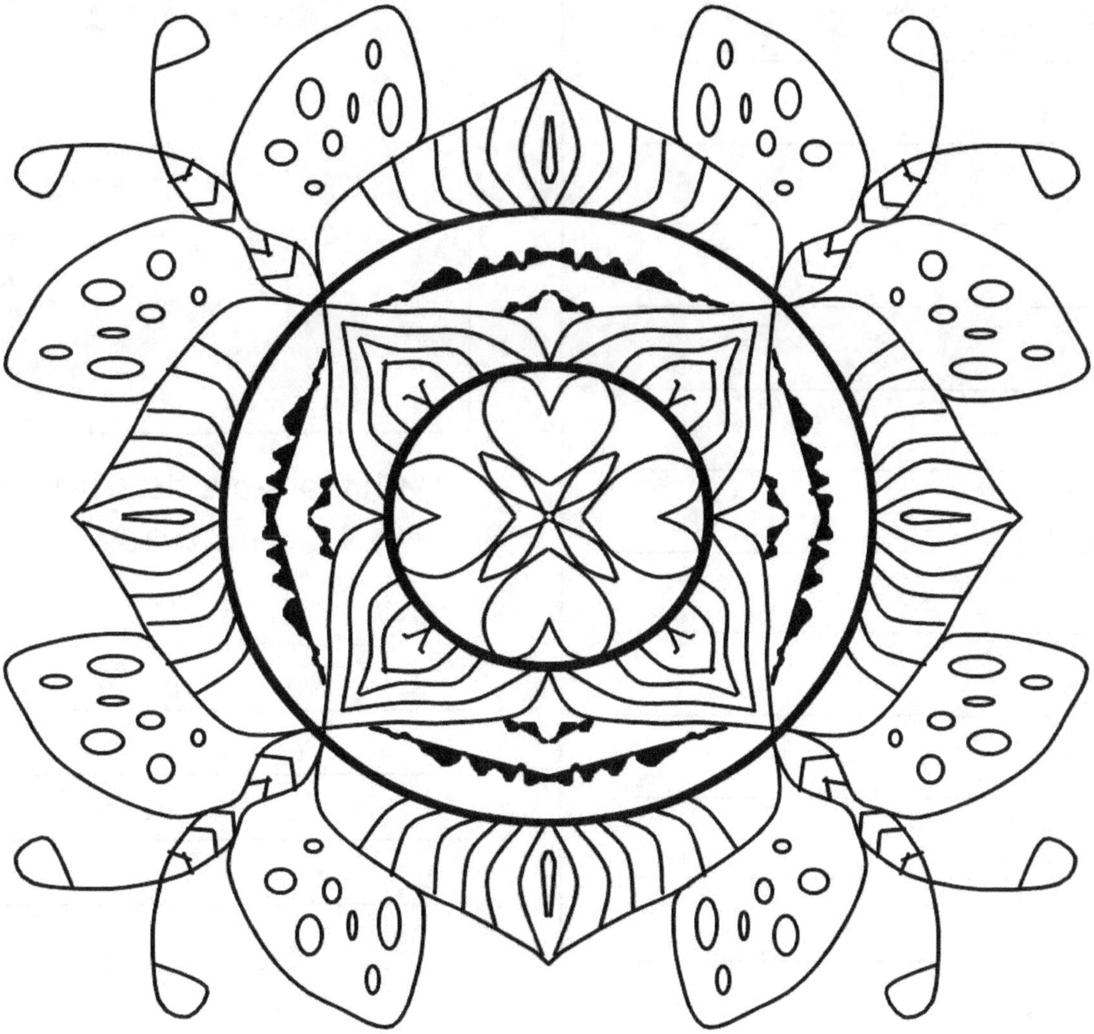

Day Thirty-five _______

5:00 _______________________

6:00 _______________________

7:00 _______________________

8:00 _______________________

9:00 _______________________

10:00 ______________________

11:00 ______________________

Noon _______________________

1:00 _______________________

2:00 _______________________

3:00 _______________________

4:00 _______________________

5:00 _______________________

6:00 _______________________

7:00 _______________________

8:00 _______________________

9:00 _______________________

10:00 ______________________

11:00 ______________________

Midnight ___________________

top priorities for today

____

____

____

____

Today's victories

Who is more determined
than you?

____

____

____

____

____

____

The *Stella Society* Workout

Exercise	Set 1	Set 2	Set 3	Set 4	Set 5	notes

Time started: _____________ Time ended: _____________

Location: ____

Feelings before training: 😊 😐 ☹️ 😜 😠 😕 😊 😎

Feelings after training 😊 😐 ☹️ 😜 😠 😕 😊 😎

NUTRITION

Meal 1

time eaten: _________

Meal 2

time eaten: _________

Meal 3

time eaten: _________

Meal 4

time eaten: _________

Meal 5

time eaten: _________

Hydration

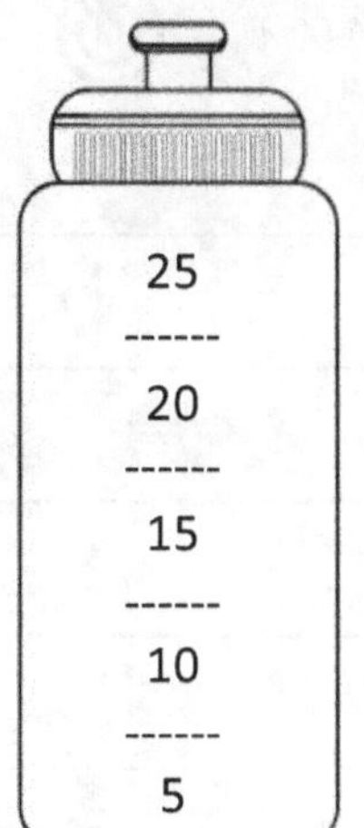

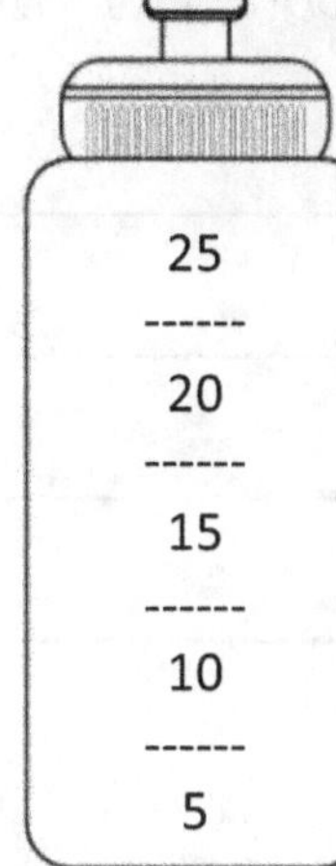

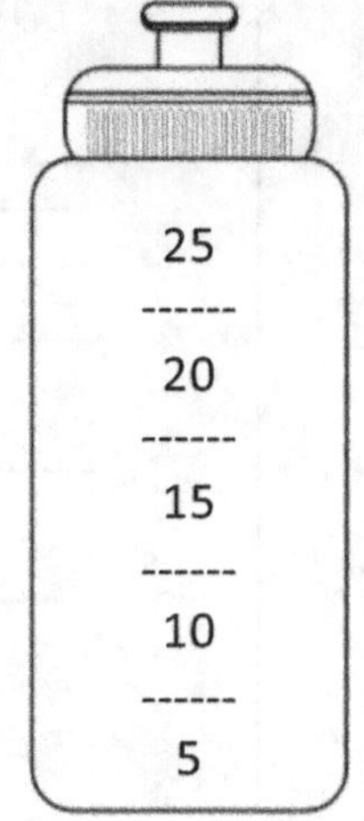

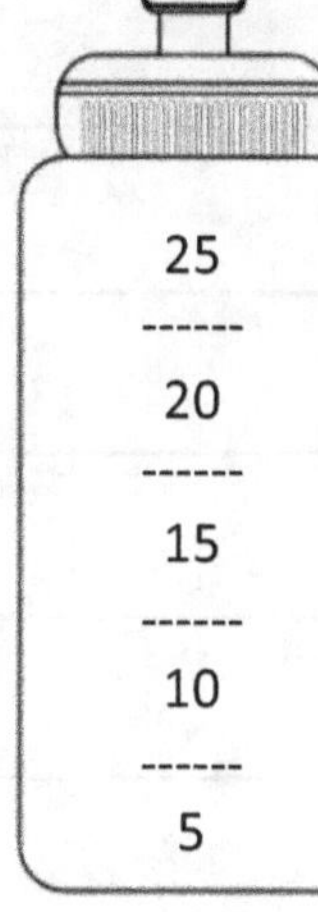

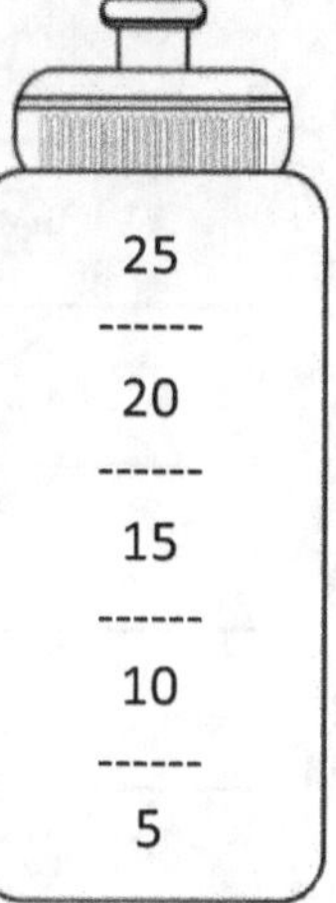

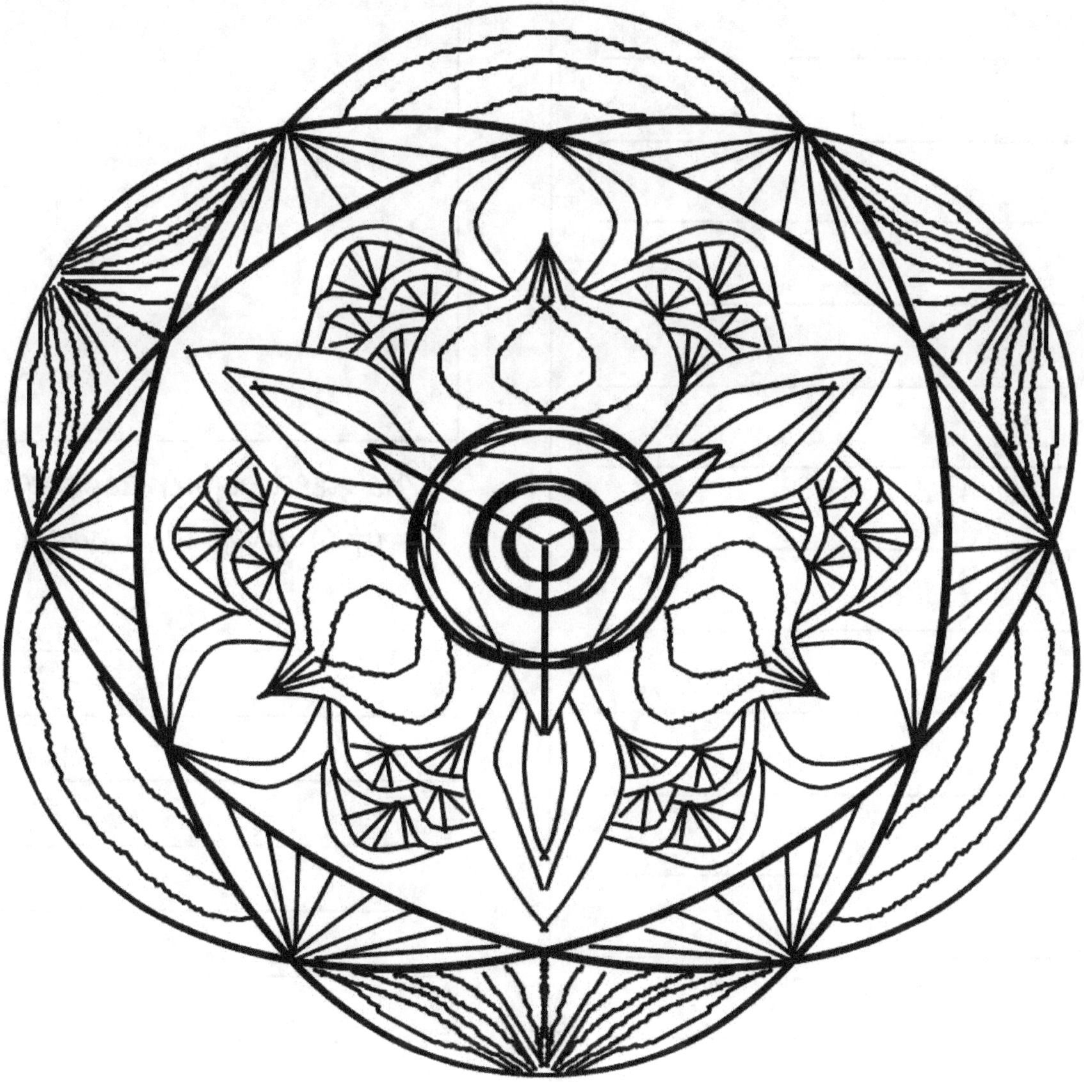

Day Thirty-six _______

5:00 _______	

5:00 _______
6:00 _______
7:00 _______
8:00 _______
9:00 _______
10:00 _______
11:00 _______
Noon _______
1:00 _______
2:00 _______
3:00 _______
4:00 _______
5:00 _______
6:00 _______
7:00 _______
8:00 _______
9:00 _______
10:00 _______
11:00 _______
Midnight _______

top priorities for today

____
____
____
____

Today's victories

Who needs your acceptance
of change and why?

____
____
____
____
____

The Stella Society Workout

Exercise	Set 1	Set 2	Set 3	Set 4	Set 5	notes

Time started: _____________ Time ended: _____________

Location: ____

Feelings before training:

Feelings after training

NUTRITION

Meal 1
time eaten: _________

Meal 2
time eaten: _________

Meal 3
time eaten: _________

Meal 4
time eaten: _________

Meal 5
time eaten: _________

Hydration

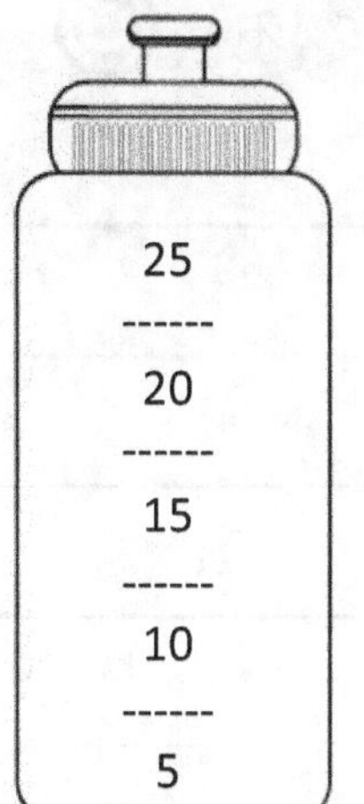

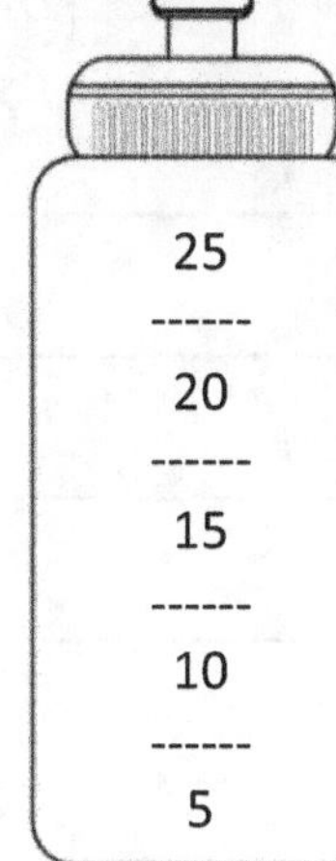

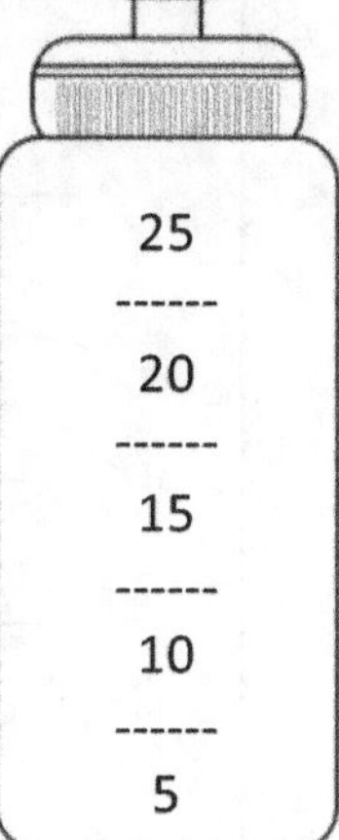

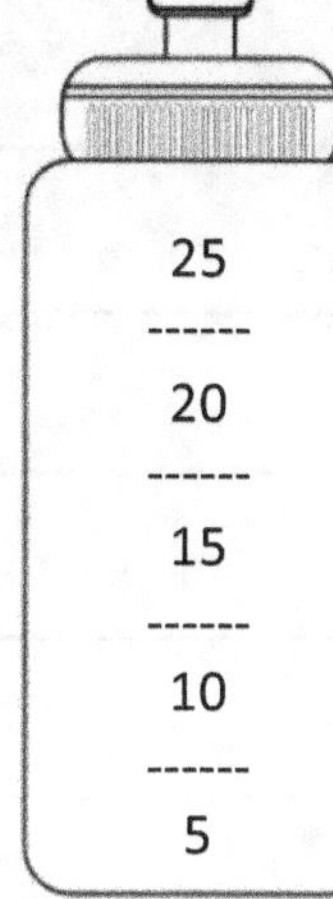

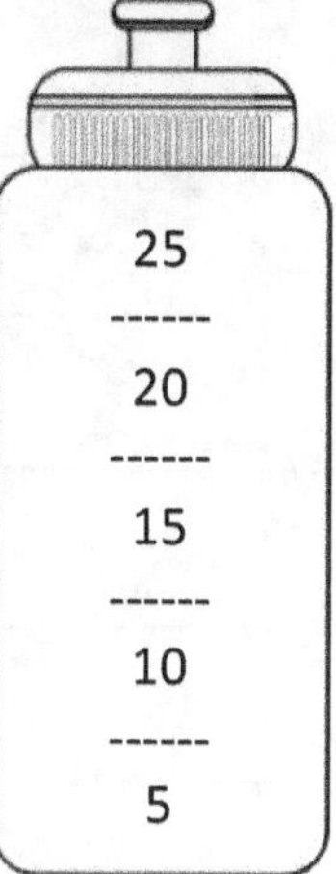

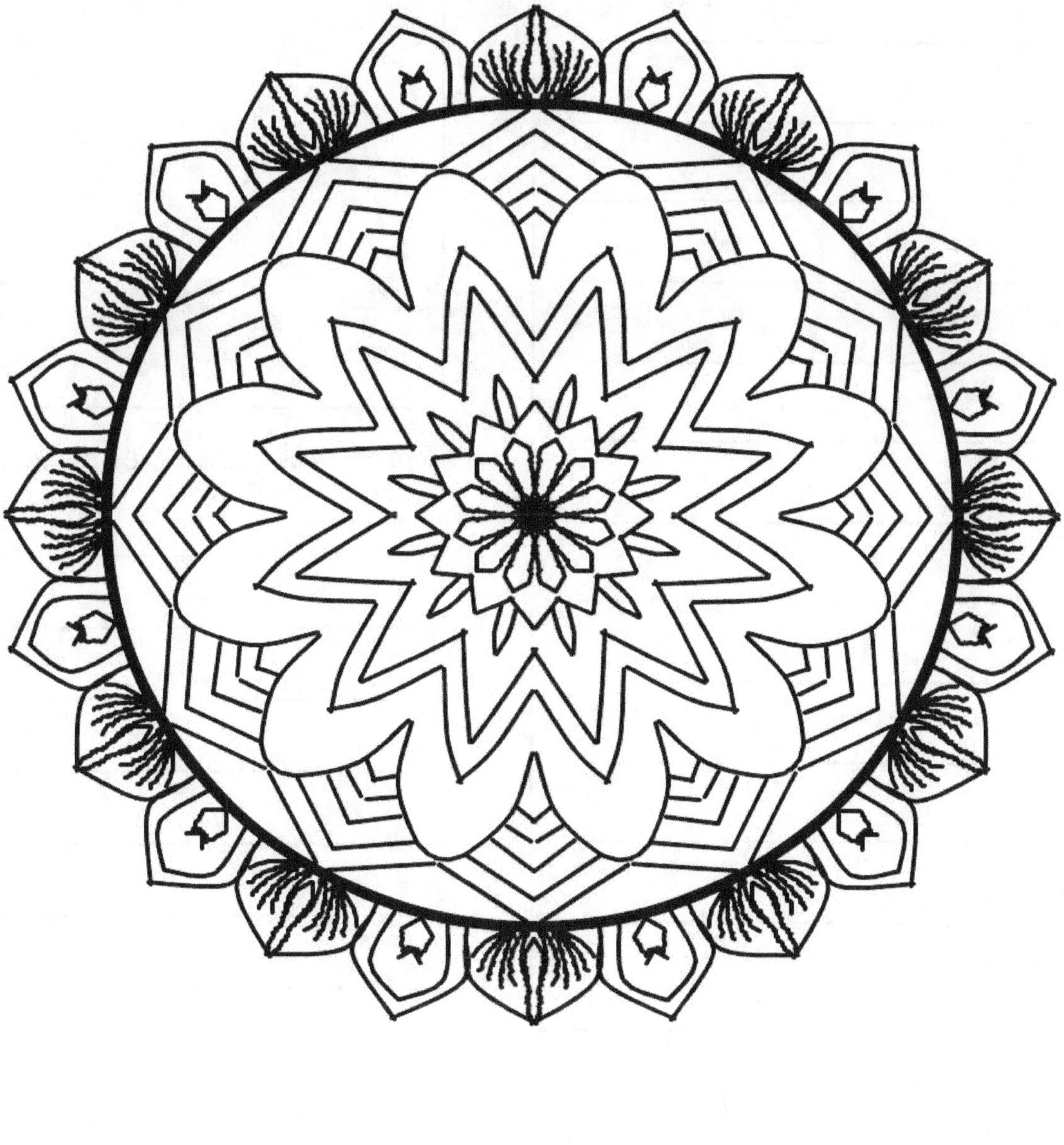

Day Thirty-seven _______

5:00 _______________________

6:00 _______________________

7:00 _______________________

8:00 _______________________

9:00 _______________________

10:00 ______________________

11:00 ______________________

Noon _______________________

1:00 _______________________

2:00 _______________________

3:00 _______________________

4:00 _______________________

5:00 _______________________

6:00 _______________________

7:00 _______________________

8:00 _______________________

9:00 _______________________

10:00 ______________________

11:00 ______________________

Midnight ___________________

top priorities for today

____

____

____

____

Today's victories

How will you be captivating?

____

____

____

____

____

____

The *Stella Society* Workout

Exercise	Set 1	Set 2	Set 3	Set 4	Set 5	notes

Time started: _____________   Time ended: _____________

Location: ____

Feelings before training:

Feelings after training

NUTRITION

Meal 1

time eaten: _________

Meal 2

time eaten: _________

Meal 3

time eaten: _________

Meal 4

time eaten: _________

Meal 5

time eaten: _________

Hydration

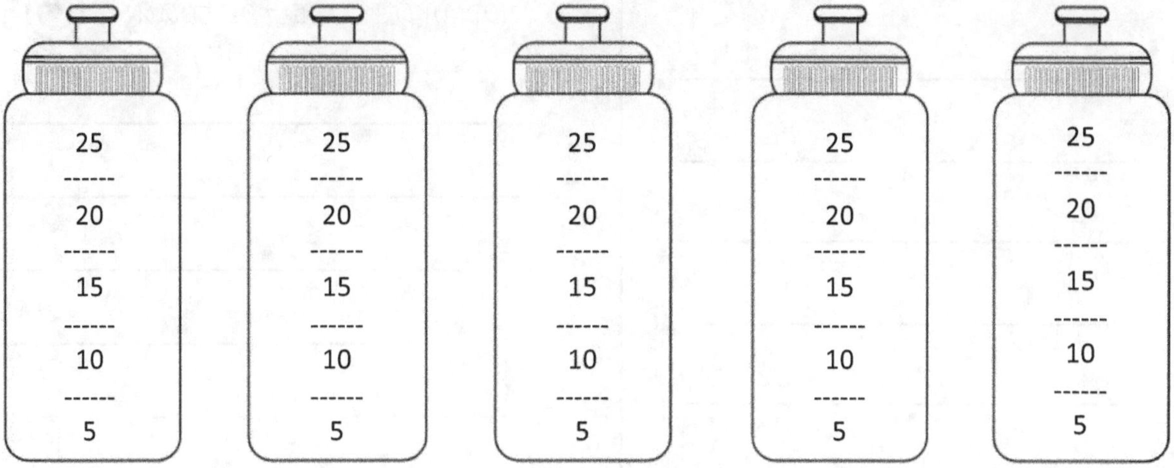

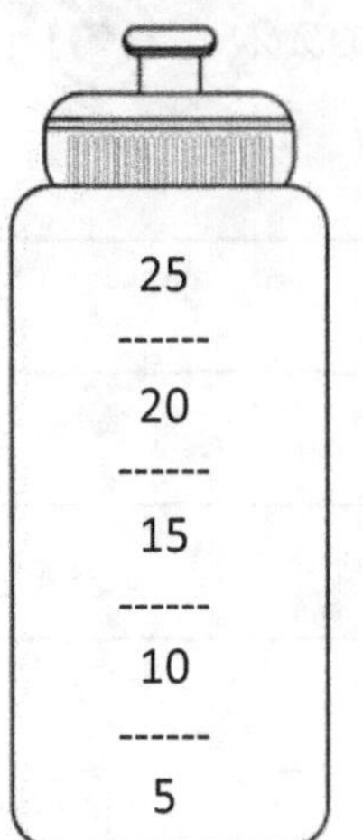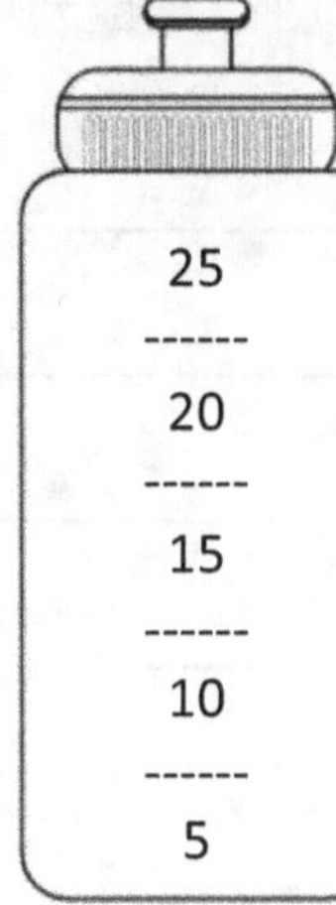

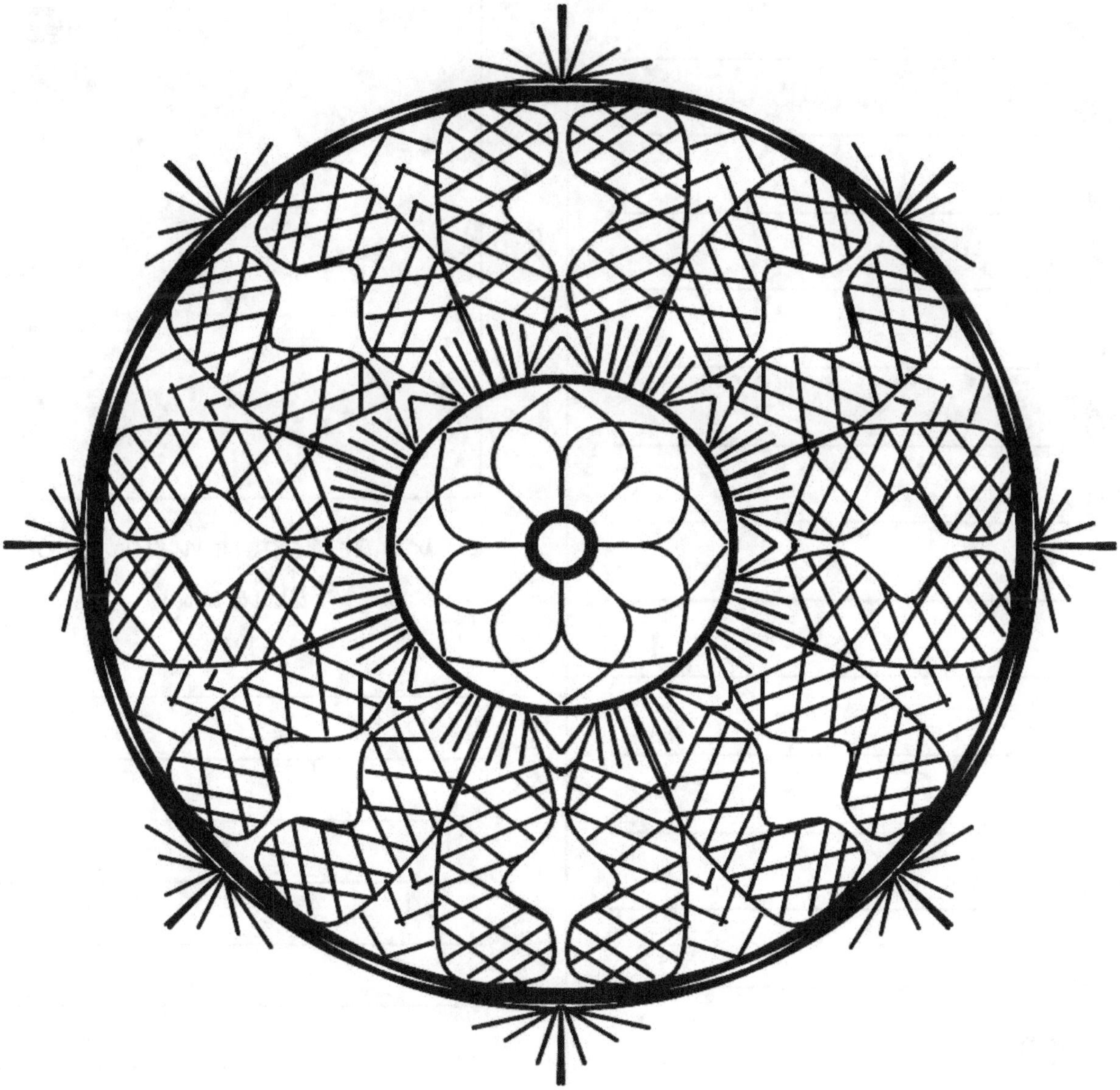

Day Thirty-eight _______

5:00 _______________________

6:00 _______________________

7:00 _______________________

8:00 _______________________

9:00 _______________________

10:00 _______________________

11:00 _______________________

Noon _______________________

1:00 _______________________

2:00 _______________________

3:00 _______________________

4:00 _______________________

5:00 _______________________

6:00 _______________________

7:00 _______________________

8:00 _______________________

9:00 _______________________

10:00 _______________________

11:00 _______________________

Midnight _______________________

top priorities for today 🎯

____

____

____

____

Today's victories 🏆

What does it mean to be alluring?

____

____

____

____

____

____

____

The 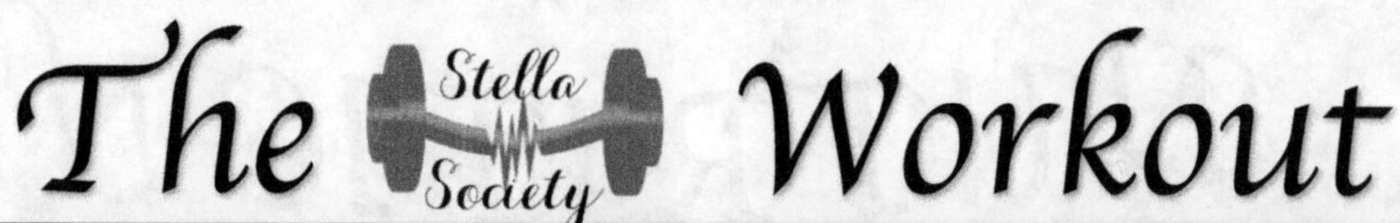 Workout

Exercise	Set 1	Set 2	Set 3	Set 4	Set 5	notes

Time started: _____________   Time ended: _____________

Location: _______________________________________

Feelings before training: ☺ 😐 ☹ 😝 😠 😟 😊 😎

Feelings after training ☺ 😐 ☹ 😝 😠 😟 😊 😎

NUTRITION

Meal 1
time eaten: _________

Meal 2
time eaten: _________

Meal 3
time eaten: _________

Meal 4
time eaten: _________

Meal 5
time eaten: _________

Hydration

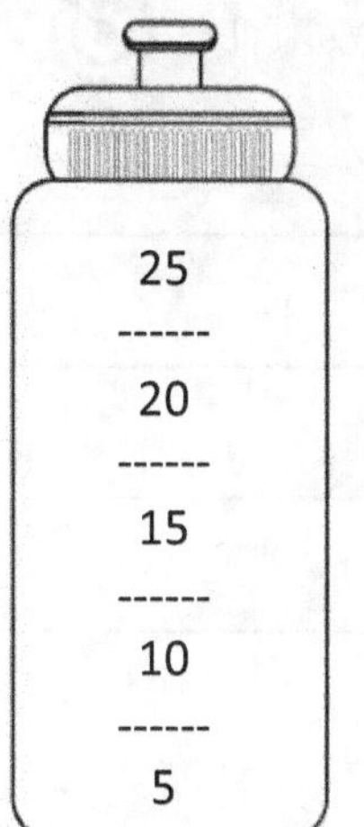

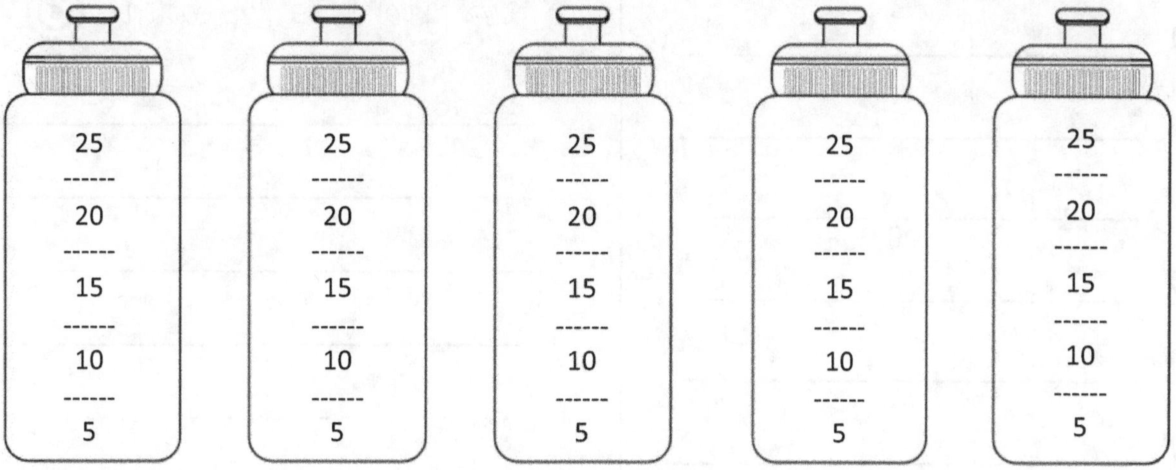

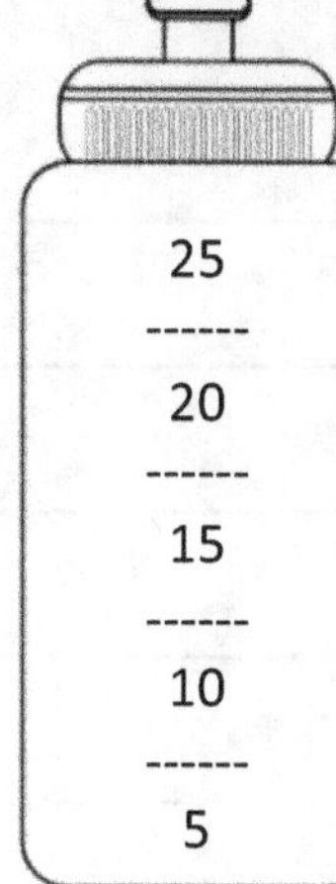

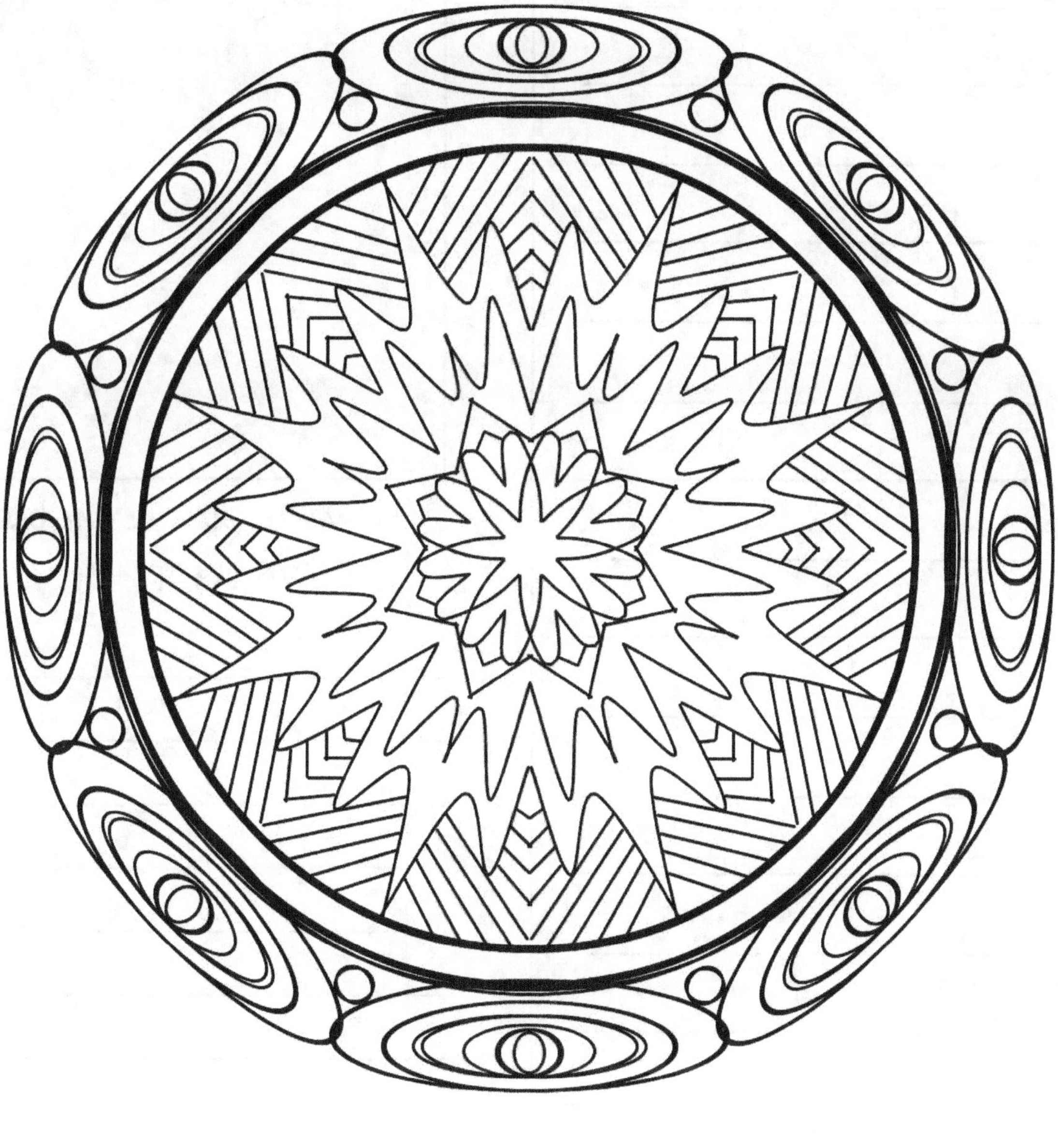

Day Thirty-nine __________

5:00 __________________________

6:00 __________________________

7:00 __________________________

8:00 __________________________

9:00 __________________________

10:00 _________________________

11:00 _________________________

Noon __________________________

1:00 __________________________

2:00 __________________________

3:00 __________________________

4:00 __________________________

5:00 __________________________

6:00 __________________________

7:00 __________________________

8:00 __________________________

9:00 __________________________

10:00 _________________________

11:00 _________________________

Midnight ______________________

top priorities for today

____

____

____

____

Today's victories

How will you be the best
version of you?

____

____

____

____

____

____

The 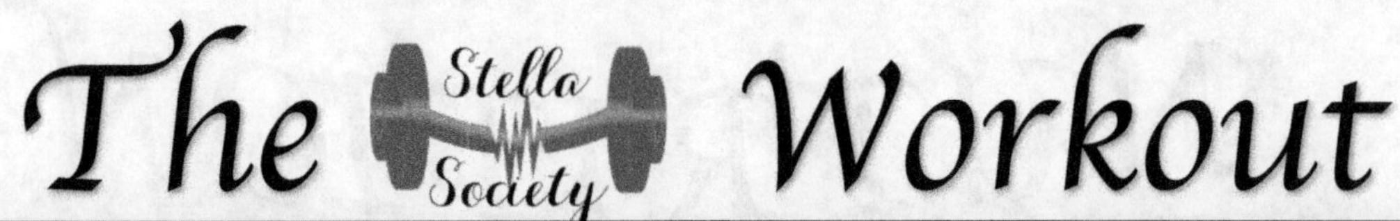 Workout

Exercise	Set 1	Set 2	Set 3	Set 4	Set 5	notes

Time started: _____________ Time ended: _____________

Location: ____

Feelings before training: 😊 😐 ☹ 😜 😠 😟 😇 😎

Feelings after training 😊 😐 ☹ 😜 😠 😟 😇 😎

NUTRITION

Meal 1

time eaten: _________

Meal 2

time eaten: _________

Meal 3

time eaten: _________

Meal 4

time eaten: _________

Meal 5

time eaten: _________

Hydration

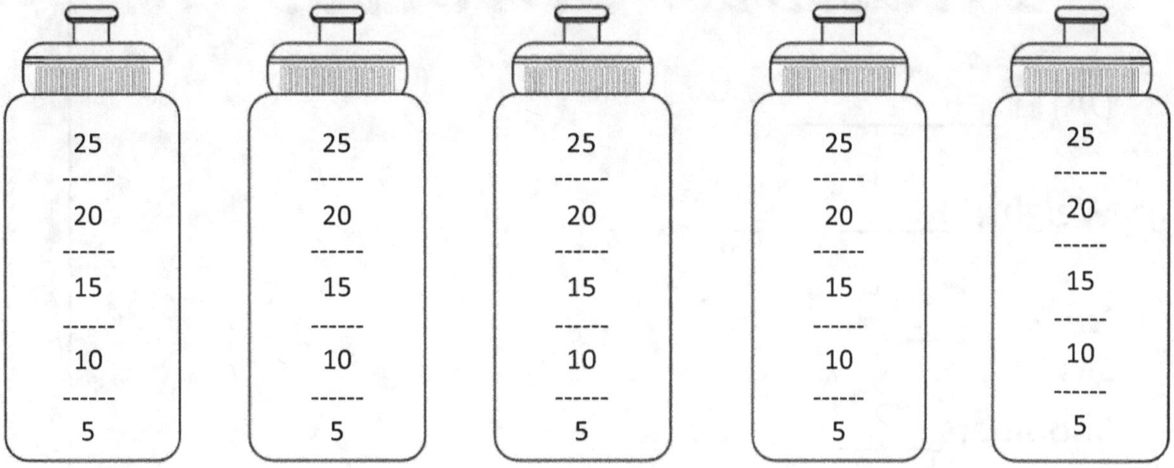

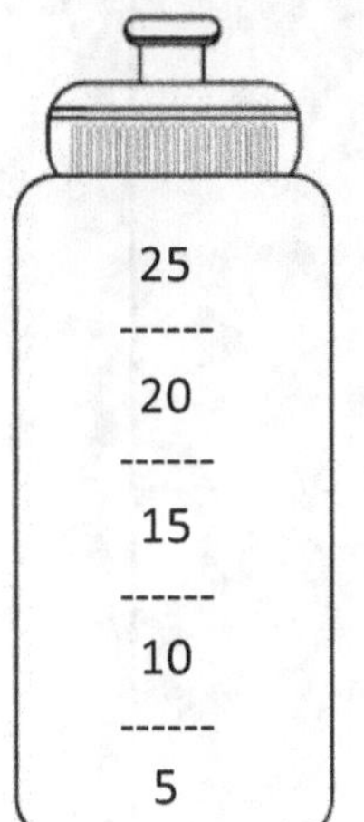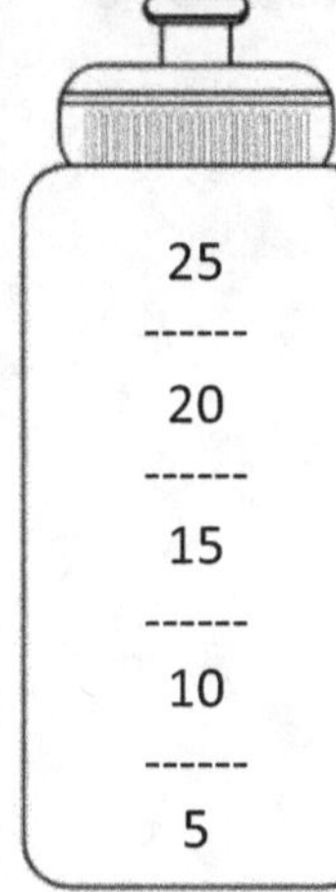

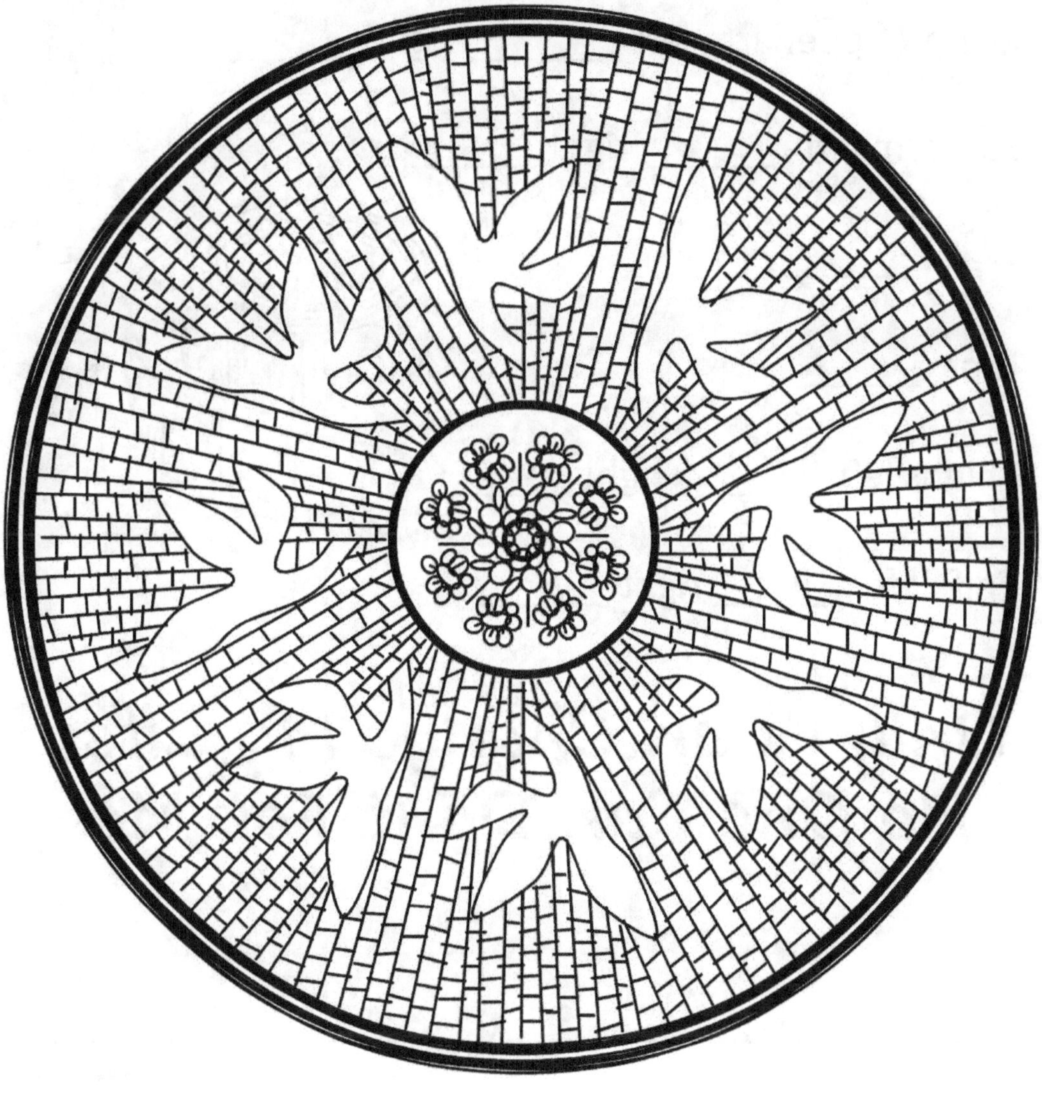

Measurements

DATE: ___________

Weight: _______

Neck _______

Shoulders _______

Chest _______

Bicep / upper arm left ________ right _______

Forearm left ________ right _______

Waist _______

Hips _______

Thighs left ________ right ________

Calf left ________ right ________

Only I Can Change My Life, No One Can Do It For Me!

Day Forty _______

5:00 ____________________

6:00 ____________________

7:00 ____________________

8:00 ____________________

9:00 ____________________

10:00 __________________

11:00 __________________

Noon ___________________

1:00 ____________________

2:00 ____________________

3:00 ____________________

4:00 ____________________

5:00 ____________________

6:00 ____________________

7:00 ____________________

8:00 ____________________

9:00 ____________________

10:00 __________________

11:00 __________________

Midnight _______________

top priorities for today

____

____

____

____

Today's victories

Do you believe in magic or miracles?

____

____

____

____

____

____

The Workout

Exercise	Set 1	Set 2	Set 3	Set 4	Set 5	notes

Time started: _____________ Time ended: _____________

Location: ____

Feelings before training:

Feelings after training

NUTRITION

Meal 1

time eaten: _________

Meal 2

time eaten: _________

Meal 3

time eaten: _________

Meal 4

time eaten: _________

Meal 5

time eaten: _________

Hydration

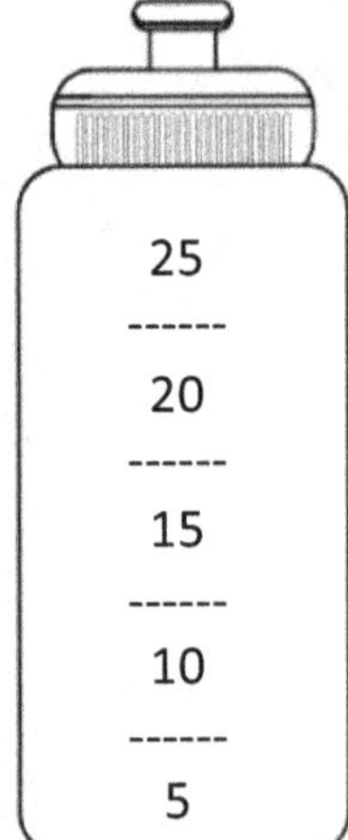
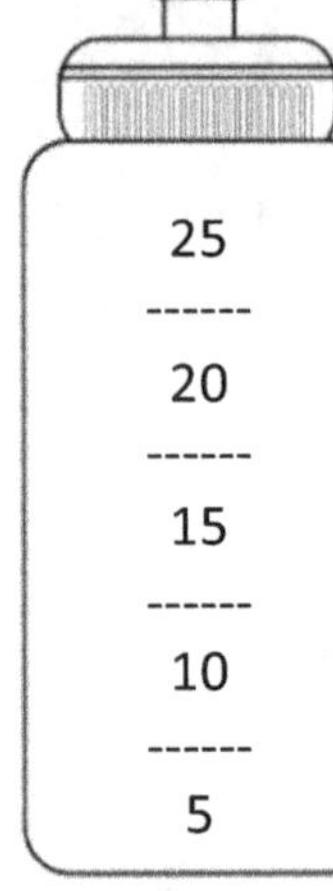
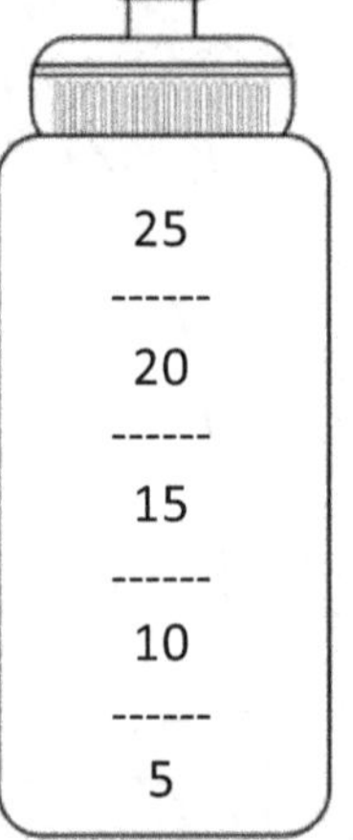
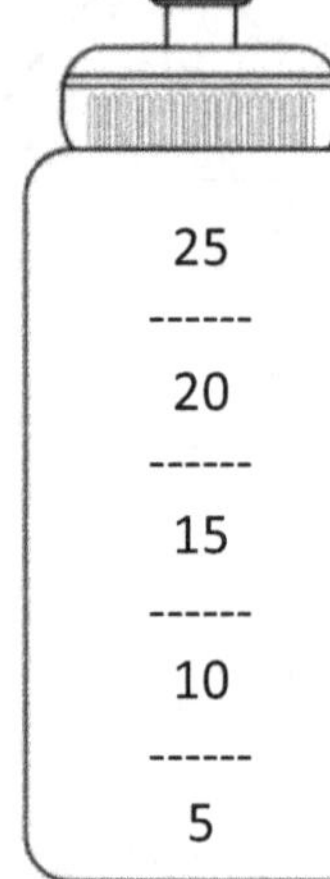
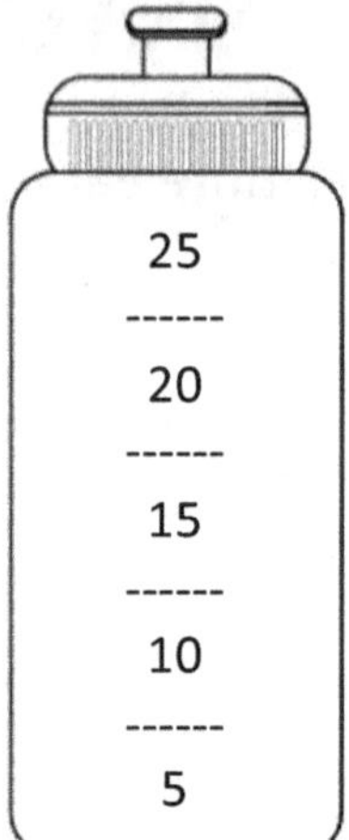

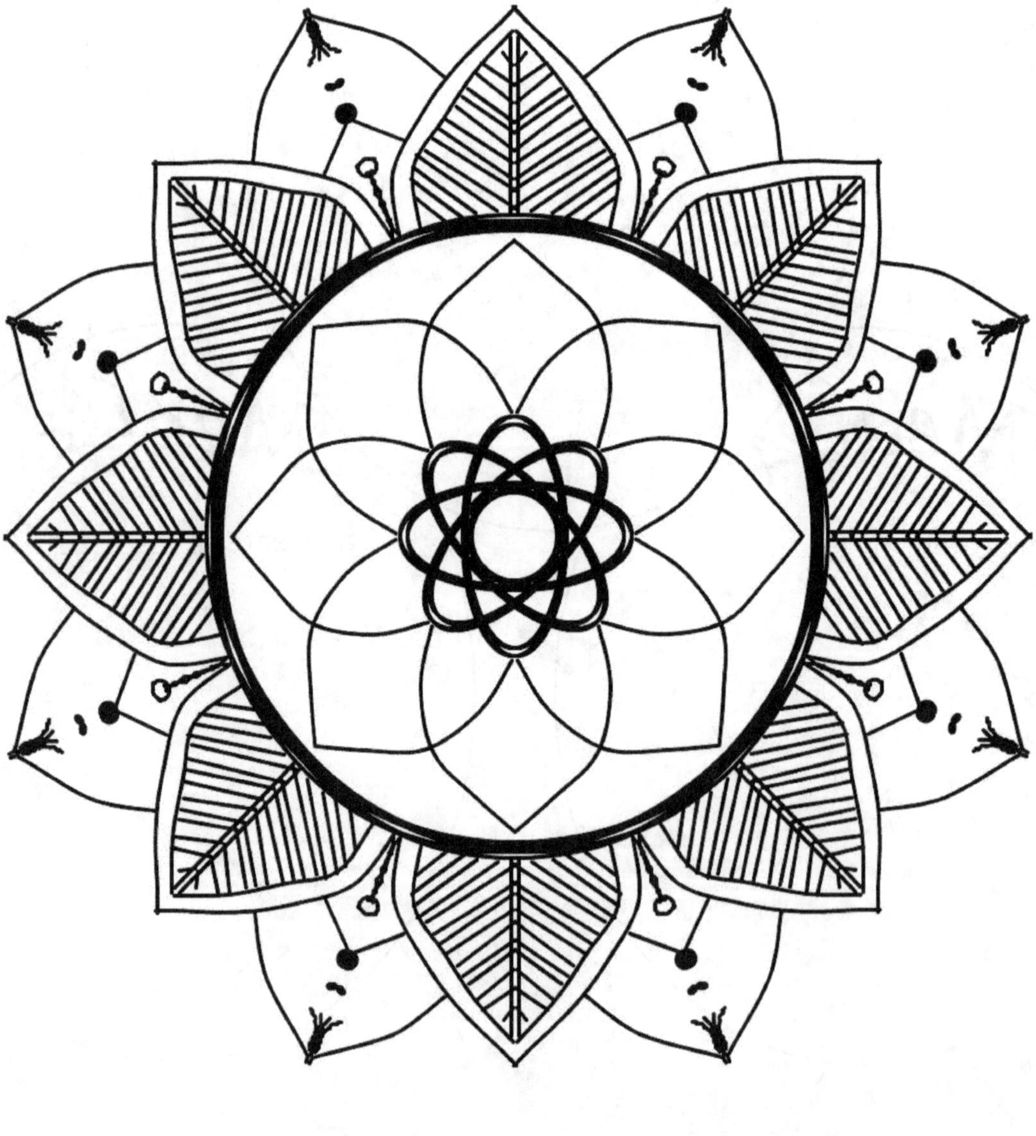

Day Forty-one _______

top priorities for today 

Today's victories

What is one thing you
want to do forever?

The *Stella Society* Workout

Exercise	Set 1	Set 2	Set 3	Set 4	Set 5	notes

Time started: _____________ Time ended: _____________

Location: ____

Feelings before training:

Feelings after training

NUTRITION

Meal 1

time eaten: _________

Meal 2

time eaten: _________

Meal 3

time eaten: _________

Meal 4

time eaten: _________

Meal 5

time eaten: _________

Hydration

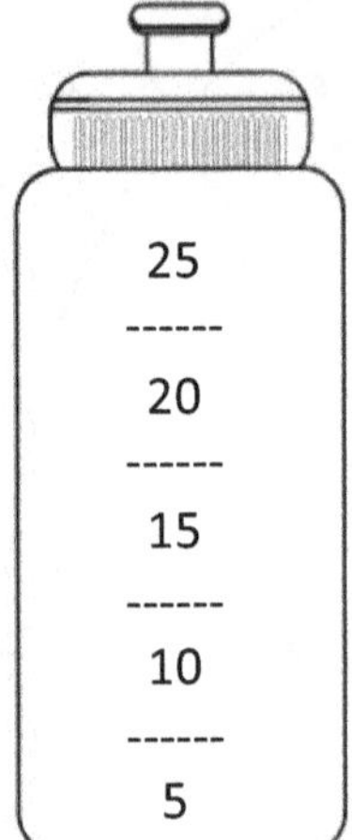

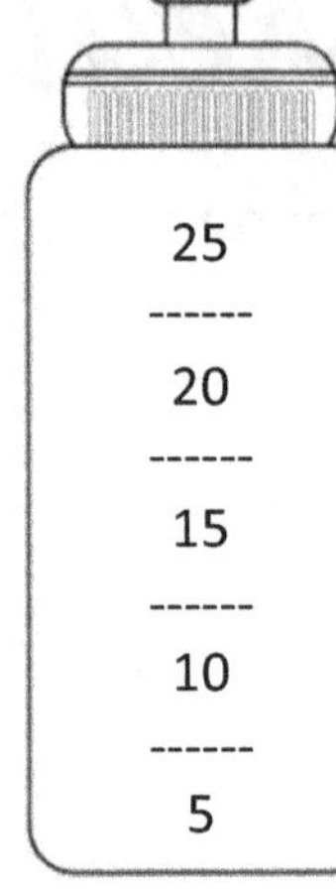

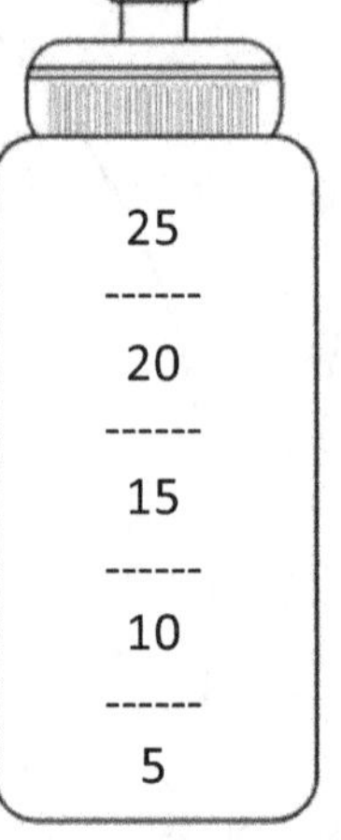

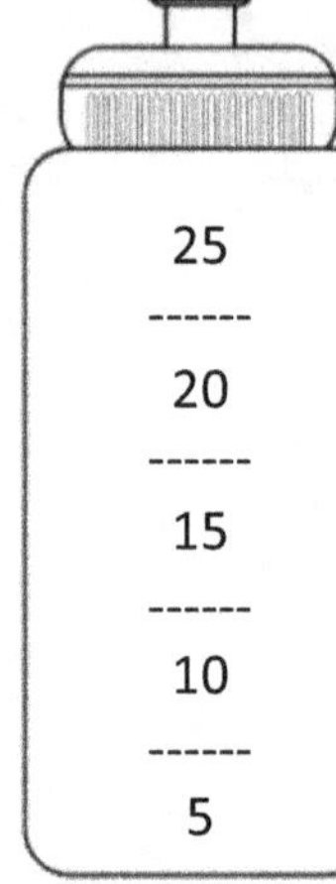

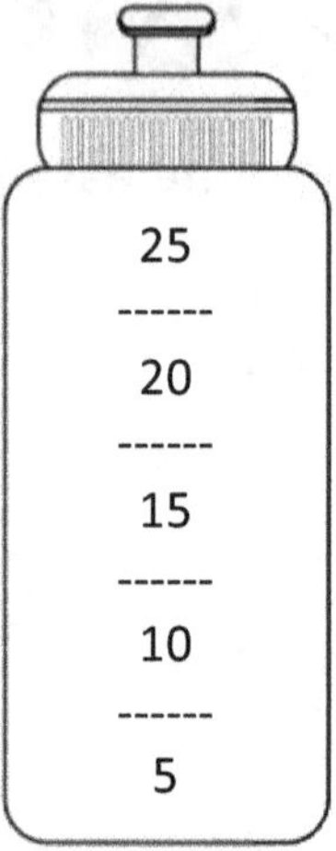

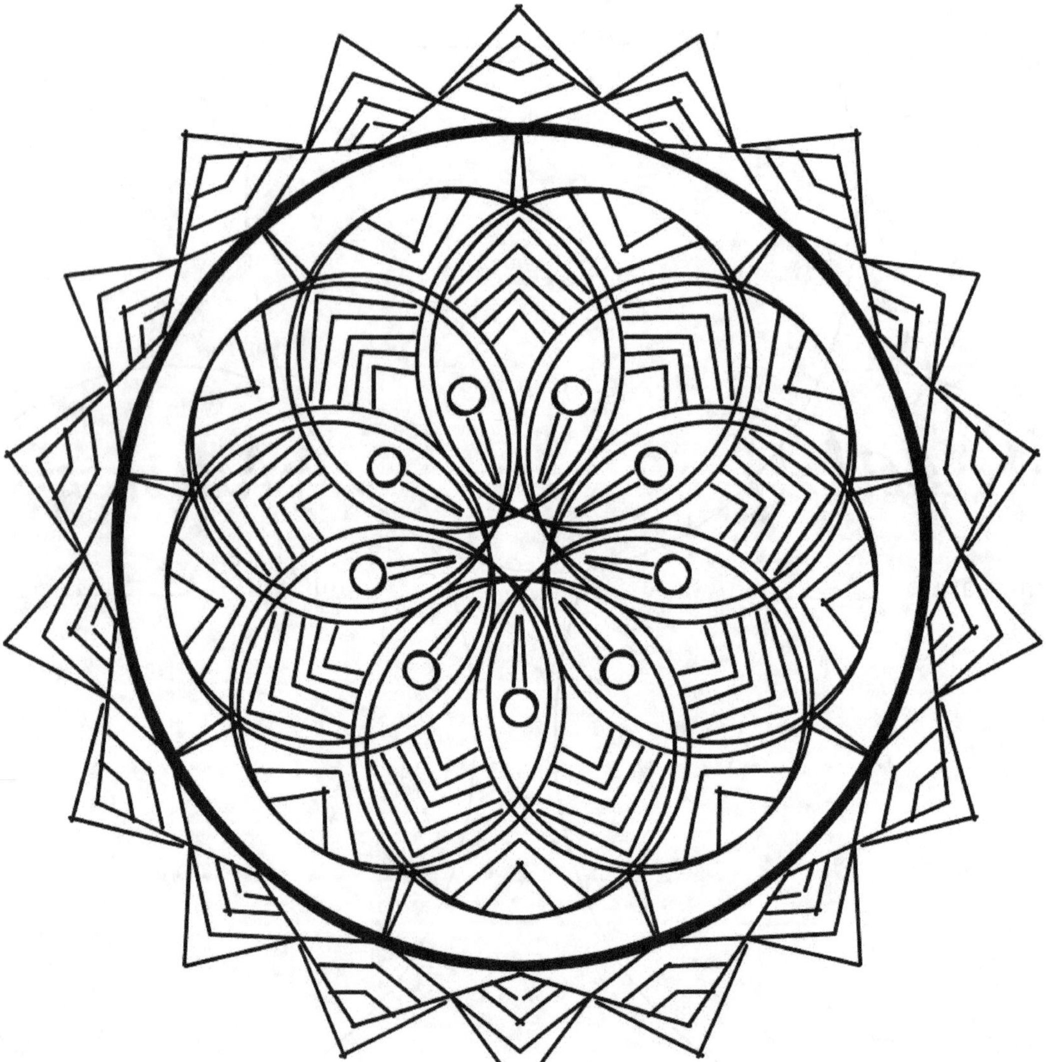

Day Forty-two _______

Time	
5:00	__________________
6:00	__________________
7:00	__________________
8:00	__________________
9:00	__________________
10:00	__________________
11:00	__________________
Noon	__________________
1:00	__________________
2:00	__________________
3:00	__________________
4:00	__________________
5:00	__________________
6:00	__________________
7:00	__________________
8:00	__________________
9:00	__________________
10:00	__________________
11:00	__________________
Midnight	__________________

Today's victories

What was your biggest victory in the last 40 days?

The Stella Society Workout

Exercise	Set 1	Set 2	Set 3	Set 4	Set 5	notes

Time started: _____________ Time ended: _____________

Location: ____

Feelings before training:

Feelings after training

NUTRITION

Meal 1
time eaten: _________

Meal 2
time eaten: _________

Meal 3
time eaten: _________

Meal 4
time eaten: _________

Meal 5
time eaten: _________

Hydration

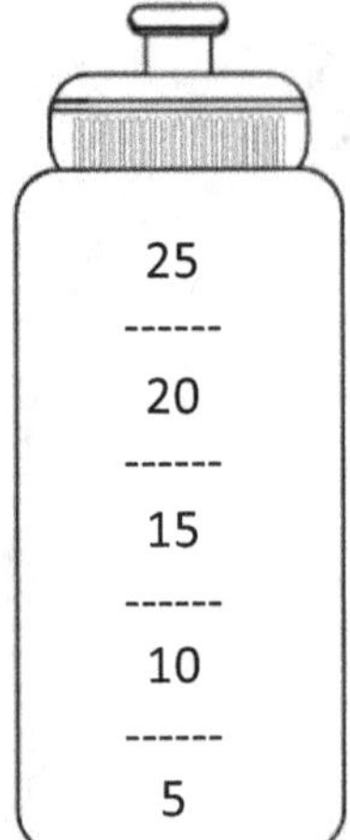

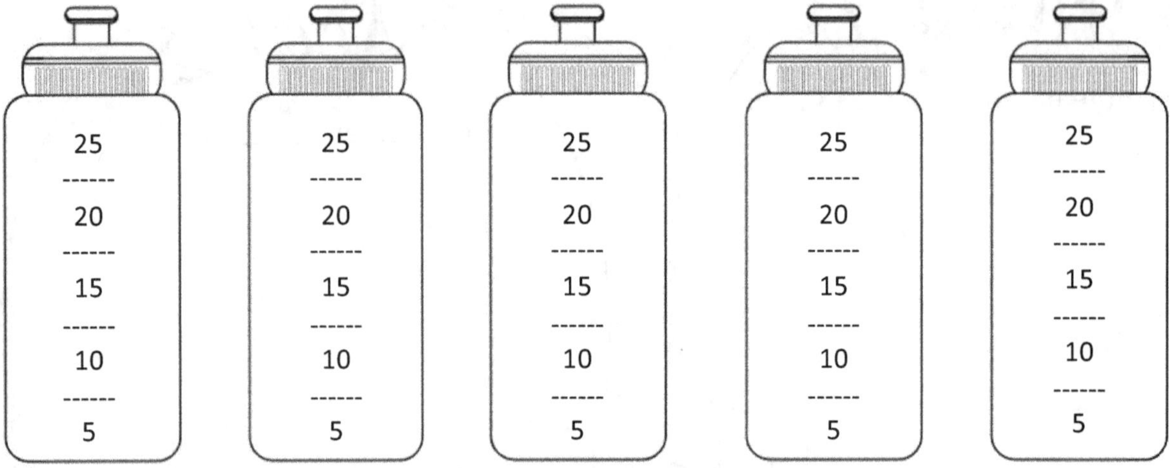

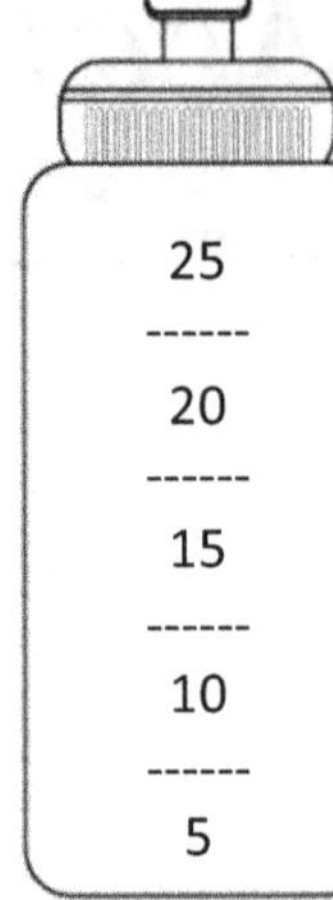

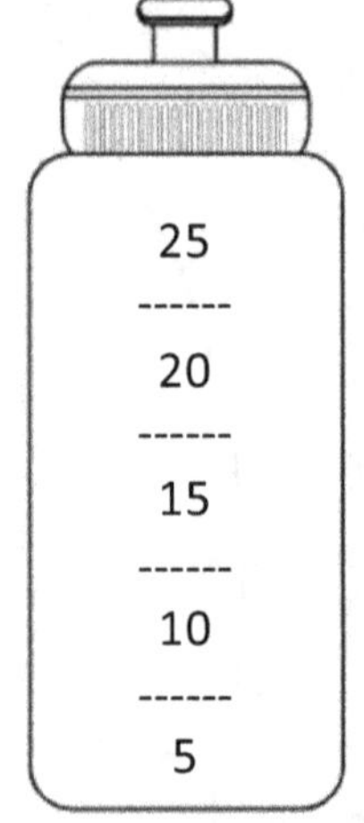

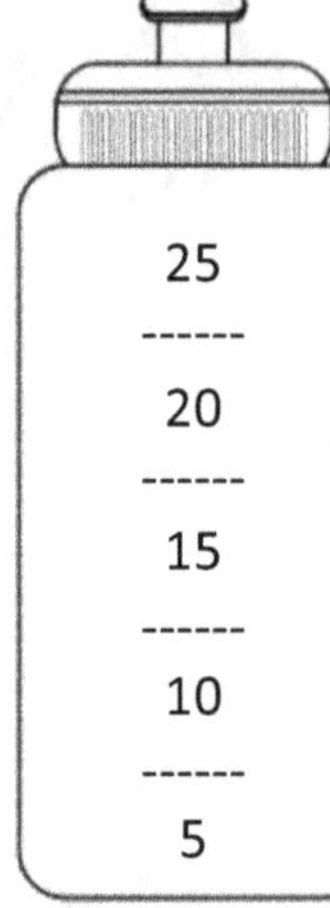

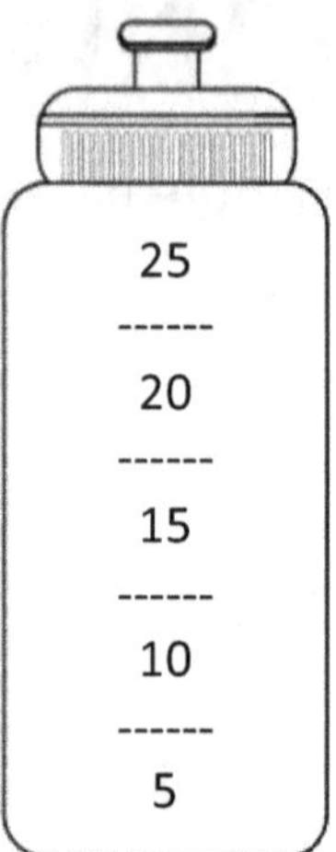

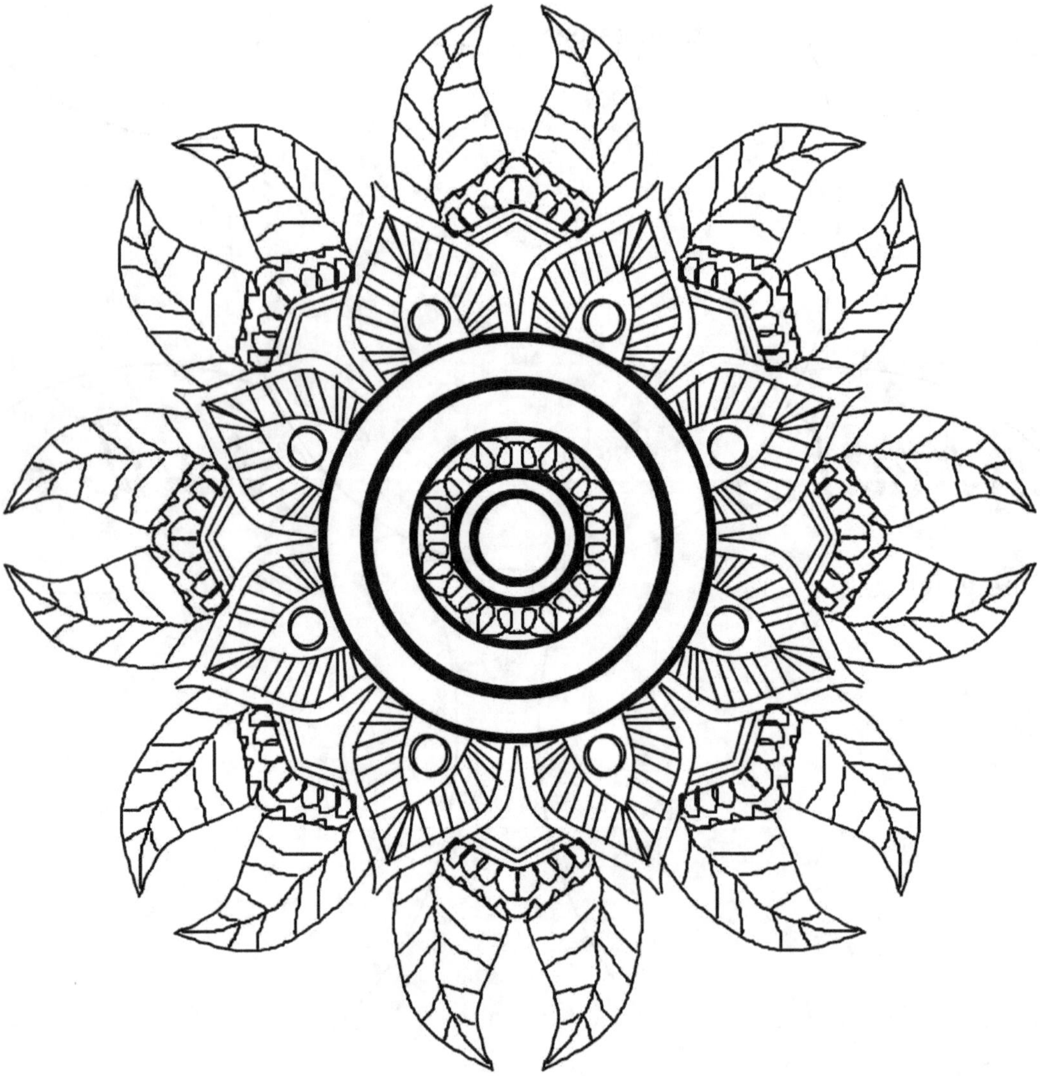

NOW WHAT?

www.ingramcontent.com/pod-product-compliance
Lightning Source LLC
Chambersburg PA
CBHW081719250726
48657CB00010B/3060